Virtual Clinical Excursions—Psychiatric

for

Keltner, Bostrom, and McGuinness:
Psychiatric Nursing,
6th Edition

Virtual Clinical Excursions—Psychiatric

for

Keltner, Bostrom, and McGuinness: Psychiatric Nursing, 6th Edition

prepared by

Susan F. McDonald, DNP, RN, PMHCNS-BC
Clinical Nurse Specialist—Inpatient Psychiatry
VA San Diego Healthcare System
San Diego, California

software developed by

Wolfsong Informatics, LLC
Tucson, Arizona

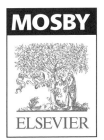

3251 Riverport Lane
Maryland Heights, Missouri 63043

VIRTUAL CLINICAL EXCURSIONS—PSYCHIATRIC FOR
KELTNER, BOSTROM, AND MCGUINNESS: PSYCHIATRIC NURSING,
SIXTH EDITION

ISBN: 978-0-323-07969-3

Copyright © 2011, 2007 by Mosby, Inc., an affiliate of Elsevier Inc.

All rights reserved. No part of this publication may be reproduced or transmitted in any form or by any means, electronic or mechanical, including photocopy, recording, or any information storage and retrieval system, without permission in writing from the publisher. Permissions may be sought directly from Elsevier's Rights Department: phone: (+1) 215 239 3804 (US) or (+44) 1865 843830 (UK); fax: (+44) 1865 853333; e-mail: healthpermissions@elsevier.com. You may also complete your request on-line via the Elsevier website at http://www.elsevier.com/permissions.

Although for mechanical reasons all pages of this publication are perforated, only those pages imprinted with an Elsevier Inc. copyright notice are intended for removal.

Notice

Knowledge and best practice in this field are constantly changing. As new research and experience broaden our knowledge, changes in practice, treatment and drug therapy may become necessary or appropriate. Readers are advised to check the most current information provided (i) on procedures featured or (ii) by the manufacturer of each product to be administered, to verify the recommended dose or formula, the method and duration of administration, and contraindications. It is the responsibility of the practitioner, relying on their own experience and knowledge of the patient, to make diagnoses, to determine dosages and the best treatment for each individual patient, and to take all appropriate safety precautions. To the fullest extent of the law, neither the Publisher nor the Authors assumes any liability for any injury and/or damage to persons or property arising out or related to any use of the material contained in this book.

ISBN: 978-0-323-07969-3

Vice President and Publisher: *Tom Wilhelm*
Editor: *Jeff Downing*
Associate Developmental Editor: *Krissy Prysmiki*
Publishing Services Manager: *Jeff Patterson*
Project Manager: *Tracey Schriefer*

Printed in the United States of America

Last digit is the print number: 9 8 7 6 5 4 3 2 1

*Workbook
prepared by*

Susan F. McDonald, DNP, RN, PMHCNS-BC
Clinical Nurse Specialist—Inpatient Psychiatry
VA San Diego Healthcare System
San Diego, California

Textbook

Norman L. Keltner, EdD, RN, APRN
Professor
School of Nursing
University of Alabama at Birmingham
Birmingham, Alabama

Carol E. Bostrom, MSN
Clinical Assistant Professor
School of Nursing
Indiana University
Indianapolis, Indiana

Teena McGuinness, PhD, CRNP, FAAN
Professor
School of Nursing
University of Alabama at Birmingham
Birmingham, Alabama

Contents

Getting Started

Getting Set Up		1
A Quick Tour		9
A Detailed Tour		24
Reducing Medication Errors		37
Lesson 1	Psychotherapeutic Management in the Continuum of Care (Chapter 2)	43
Lesson 2	The Nurse-Patient Relationship (Chapters 6 and 7)	51
Lesson 3	Nursing Process (Chapter 8)	59
Lesson 4	Stress, Anxiety, Coping, and Crisis (Chapter 9)	67
Lesson 5	Cultural Competence and Spirituality (Chapters 14 and 15)	75
Lesson 6	Schizophrenia (Chapter 27)	85
Lesson 7	Depression (Chapter 28)	97
Lesson 8	Anxiety Disorders (Chapter 30)	107
Lesson 9	Cognitive Disorders (Chapter 31)	113
Lesson 10	Substance-Related Disorders (Chapter 34)	125
Lesson 11	Eating Disorders (Chapter 36)	135
Lesson 12	Nutraceuticals and Mental Health (Chapter 38)	145
Lesson 13	Survivors of Violence and Trauma (Chapter 39)	153
Lesson 14	The Adolescent Patient (Chapter 40)	165
Lesson 15	Mental Disorders in Older Adults (Chapter 41)	171

Table of Contents
Keltner: Psychiatric Nursing, 6th Edition

1. Introduction to Psychiatric Nursing
2. Psychotherapeutic Management in the Continuum of Care (Lesson 1)
3. Models for Working with Psychiatric Patients
4. Legal Issues
5. Psychobiologic Bases of Behavior
6. Nurse-Patient Communication (Lesson 2)
7. Nurse-Patient Relationship (Lesson 2)
8. Nursing Process (Lesson 3)
9. Anxiety, Coping, and Crisis (Lesson 4)
10. Suicide and Other Self-Destructive Behaviors
11. Working with the Aggressive Patient
12. Working with Groups of Patients
13. Working with the Family
14. Cultural Competence in Psychiatric Nursing (Lesson 5)
15. Spirituality (Lesson 5)
16. Introduction to Psychotropic Drugs
17. Antiparkinsonian Drugs
18. Antipsychotic Drugs
19. Antidepressant Drugs
20. Antimanic Drugs
21. Antianxiety Drugs
22. Antidementia Drugs
23. Introduction to Milieu Management
24. Variables Affecting the Therapeutic Environment
25. Therapeutic Environment in Various Treatment Settings
26. Introduction to Psychopathology
27. Schizophrenia and Other Psychoses (Lesson 6)
28. Depression (Lesson 7)
29. Bipolar Disorders
30. Anxiety-Related, Somatoform, and Dissociative Disorders (Lesson 8)
31. Cognitive Disorders (Lesson 9)
32. Personality Disorders
33. Sexual Disorders
34. Substance-Related Disorders (Lesson 10)
35. Dual Diagnosis
36. Eating Disorders (Lesson 11)
37. Behavior and Somatic Therapies
38. Nutraceuticals and Mental Health (Lesson 12)
39. Survivors of Violence and Trauma (Lesson 13)
40. Child and Adolescent Psychiatric Nursing (Lesson 14)
41. Mental Disorders in Older Adults (Lesson 15)
42. War-Related Psychiatric Disorders in Soldiers

Appendices

Diagnostic Criteria for Mental Disorders (DSM-IV-TR)
North American Nursing Diagnosis Association–Approved Nursing Diagnoses, 2005-2006

Glossary

Index

Getting Started

GETTING SET UP

■ MINIMUM SYSTEM REQUIREMENTS

WINDOWS®

Windows Vista®, XP, 2000 (Recommend Windows XP/2000)
Pentium® III processor (or equivalent) @ 600 MHz (Recommend 800 MHz or better)
256 MB of RAM (Recommend 1 GB or more for Windows Vista)
800 x 600 screen size (Recommend 1024 x 768)
Thousands of colors
12x CD-ROM drive

Note: Windows Vista and XP require administrator privileges for installation.

MACINTOSH®

MAC OS X (up to 10.6.1)
Apple Power PC G3 @ 500 MHz or better
128 MB of RAM (Recommend 256 MB or more)
800 x 600 screen size (Recommend 1024 x 768)
Thousands of colors
12x CD-ROM drive
Stereo speakers or headphones

2 GETTING STARTED

■ INSTALLATION INSTRUCTIONS

WINDOWS

1. Insert the *Virtual Clinical Excursions—Psychiatric* CD-ROM.
2. The setup screen should appear automatically if the current product is not already installed. Windows Vista users may be asked to authorize additional security prompts.
3. Follow the onscreen instructions during the setup process.

   If the setup screen does *not* appear automatically (and *Virtual Clinical Excursions—Psychiatric* has not been installed already):
   a. Click the **My Computer** icon on your desktop or on your Start menu.
   b. Double-click on your CD-ROM drive.
   c. If installation does not start at this point:
      (1) Click the **Start** icon on the taskbar and select the **Run** option.
      (2) Type d:\setup.exe (where "d:\" is your CD-ROM drive) and press **OK**.
      (3) Follow the onscreen instructions for installation.

MACINTOSH

1. Insert the *Virtual Clinical Excursions—Psychiatric* CD in the CD-ROM drive. The disk icon will appear on your desktop.
2. Double-click on the disk icon.
3. Double-click on the VCEPSYCH_MAC run file.

Note: Virtual Clinical Excursions—Psychiatric for Macintosh does not have an installation setup and can only be run directly from the CD.

■ HOW TO USE VIRTUAL CLINICAL EXCURSIONS—PSYCHIATRIC

WINDOWS

1. Double-click on the *Virtual Clinical Excursions—Psychiatric* icon located on your desktop.
2. Or navigate to the program via the Windows Start menu.

Note: If your computer uses Windows Vista, right-click on the desktop shortcut and choose **Properties**. In the Compatibility Mode, check the box for "Run as Administrator." Below is a screen capture to show what this looks like.

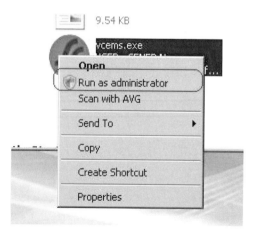

Copyright © 2011, 2007 by Mosby, Inc., an affiliate of Elsevier Inc. All rights reserved.

MACINTOSH

1. Insert the *Virtual Clinical Excursions—Psychiatric* CD in the CD-ROM drive. The disk icon will appear on your desktop.
2. Double-click on the disk icon.
3. Double-click on the VCEPSYCH_MAC run file.

■ SCREEN SETTINGS

For best results, your computer monitor resolution should be set at a minimum of 800 x 600. The number of colors displayed should be set to "thousands or higher" (High Color or 16 bit) or "millions of colors" (True Color or 24 bit).

Windows

1. From the **Start** menu, select **Control Panel** (on some systems, you will first go to **Settings**, then to **Control Panel**).
2. Double-click on the **Display** icon.
3. Click on the **Settings** tab.
4. Under **Screen resolution** use the slider bar to select **800 by 600 pixels**.
5. Access the **Colors** drop-down menu by clicking on the down arrow.
6. Select **High Color (16 bit)** or **True Color (24 bit)**.
7. Click on **OK**.
8. You may be asked to verify the setting changes. Click **Yes**.
9. You may be asked to restart your computer to accept the changes. Click **Yes**.

Macintosh

1. Select the **Monitors** control panel.
2. Select **800 x 600** (or similar) from the **Resolution** area.
3. Select **Thousands** or **Millions** from the **Color Depth** area.

■ WEB BROWSERS

Supported web browsers include Microsoft Internet Explorer (IE) version 6.0 or higher, Netscape version 7.1 or higher, and Mozilla version 1.4 or higher.

If you use America Online® (AOL) for web access, you will need AOL version 4.0 or higher and one of the browsers listed above. Do not use earlier versions of AOL with earlier versions of IE, because you will have difficulty accessing many features.

For best results with AOL:
- Connect to the Internet using AOL version 4.0 or higher.
- Open a private chat within AOL (this allows the AOL client to remain open, without asking whether you wish to disconnect while minimized).
- Minimize AOL.
- Launch a recommended browser.

TECHNICAL SUPPORT

Technical support for this product is available 24 hours a day, seven days a week, excluding holidays. Before calling, be sure that your computer meets the minimum system requirements to run this software. Inside the United States and Canada, call 1-800-692-9010. Outside North America, call 314-447-8094. You may also fax your questions to 314-447-8078 or contact Technical Support through e-mail: technical.support@elsevier.com.

Trademarks: Windows, Macintosh, Pentium, and America Online are registered trademarks.

Copyright © 2011, 2007 by Mosby, Inc., an affiliate of Elsevier Inc.

All rights reserved. No part of this product may be reproduced or transmitted in any form or by any means, electronic or mechanical, including input or storage in any information system, without written permission from the publisher.

ACCESSING *Virtual Clinical Excursions—Psychiatric* FROM EVOLVE

The product you have purchased is part of the Evolve family of online courses and learning resources. Please read the following information thoroughly to get started.

To access your instructor's course on Evolve:

Your instructor will provide you with the username and password needed to access this specific course on the Evolve Learning System. Once you have received this information, please follow these instructions:

1. Go to the Evolve student page (http://evolve.elsevier.com/student).

2. Enter your username and password in the **Login to My Evolve** area and click the **Login** button.

3. You will be taken to your personalized **My Evolve** page, where the course will be listed in the **My Courses** module.

TECHNICAL REQUIREMENTS

To use an Evolve course, you will need access to a computer that is connected to the Internet and equipped with web browser software that supports frames. For optimal performance, it is recommended that you have speakers and use a high-speed Internet connection. However, slower dial-up modems (56 K minimum) are acceptable.

Whichever browser you use, the browser preferences must be set to enable cookies and the cache must be set to reload every time.

Enable Cookies

Browser	Steps
Internet Explorer (IE) 6.0 or higher	1. Select **Tools → Internet Options**. 2. Select **Privacy** tab. 3. Use the slider (slide down) to **Accept All Cookies**. 4. Click **OK**. -OR- 3. Click the **Advanced** button. 4. Click the check box next to **Override Automatic Cookie Handling**. 5. Click the **Accept** radio buttons under **First-party Cookies** and **Third-party Cookies**. 6. Click **OK**.
Mozilla Firefox 2.0 or higher	1. Select **Tools → Options**. 2. Select the **Privacy** icon. 3. Click to expand Cookies. 4. Select **Allow sites to set cookies**. 5. Click **OK**.

Set Cache to Always Reload a Page

Browser	Steps
Internet Explorer (IE) 6.0 or higher	1. Select **Tools → Internet Options**. 2. Select **General** tab. 3. Go to the **Temporary Internet Files** and click the **Settings** button. 4. Select the radio button for **Every visit to the page** and click **OK** when complete.
Mozilla Firefox 2.0 or higher	1. Select **Tools → Options**. 2. Select the **Privacy** icon. 3. Click to expand Cache. 4. Set the value to "0" in the **Use up to: __ MB of disk space for the cache** field. 5. Click **OK**.

Copyright © 2011, 2007 by Mosby, Inc., an affiliate of Elsevier Inc. All rights reserved.

Plug-Ins

Adobe Acrobat Reader—With the free Acrobat Reader software, you can view and print Adobe PDF files. Many Evolve products offer student and instructor manuals, checklists, and more in this format!

Download at: http://www.adobe.com

Apple QuickTime—Install this to hear word pronunciations, heart and lung sounds, and many other helpful audio clips within Evolve Online Courses!

Download at: http://www.apple.com

Adobe Flash Player—This player will enhance your viewing of many Evolve web pages, as well as educational short-form to long-form animation within the Evolve Learning System!

Download at: http://www.adobe.com

Adobe Shockwave Player—Shockwave is best for viewing the many interactive learning activities within Evolve Online Courses!

Download at: http://www.adobe.com

Microsoft Word Viewer—With this viewer, Microsoft Word users can share documents with those who don't have Word, and users without Word can open and view Word documents. Many Evolve products have testbank, student and instructor manuals, and other documents available for downloading and viewing on your own computer!

Download at: http://www.microsoft.com

Microsoft PowerPoint Viewer—With this viewer, you can access PowerPoint 97, 2000, and 2002 presentations even if you don't have PowerPoint. Many Evolve products have slides available for downloading and viewing on your own computer!

Download at: http://www.microsoft.com

Copyright © 2011, 2007 by Mosby, Inc., an affiliate of Elsevier Inc. All rights reserved.

SUPPORT INFORMATION

Live phone support is available to customers in the United States and Canada at **800-401-9962** 24 hours a day, seven days a week. Support is also available through email at evolve-support@elsevier.com.

Online 24/7 support can be accessed on the Evolve website (http://evolve.elsevier.com). Resources include:

- Guided tours
- Tutorials
- Frequently asked questions (FAQs)
- Online copies of course user guides
- And much more!

A QUICK TOUR

Welcome to *Virtual Clinical Excursions—Psychiatric*, a virtual hospital setting in which you can work with multiple complex patient simulations and also learn to access and evaluate the information resources that are essential for high-quality patient care. The virtual hospital, Pacific View Regional Hospital, has realistic architecture and access to patient rooms, a Nurses' Station, and a Medication Room.

■ BEFORE YOU START

Make sure you have your textbook nearby when you use the *Virtual Clinical Excursions—Psychiatric* CD. You will want to consult topic areas in your textbook frequently while working with the CD and using this workbook.

■ HOW TO SIGN IN

- Enter your name on the Student Nurse identification badge.
- Next, click the down arrow next to **Select Floor**. This drop-down menu lists only the floors on which there are currently patients with psychiatric nursing needs: Medical-Surgical, Obstetrics, Pediatrics, and Skilled Nursing. (For this quick tour, choose **Obstetrics**.)
- Now choose one of the four periods of care in which to work. In Periods of Care 1 through 3, you can actively engage in patient assessment, entry of data in the electronic patient record (EPR), and medication administration. Period of Care 4 presents the day in review. Highlight and click the appropriate period of care. (For this quick tour, choose **Period of Care 1: 0730-0815**.)
- Click **Go**. This takes you to the Patient List screen (see example on page 11). Note that the virtual time is provided in the box at the lower left corner of the screen (0730, since we chose Period of Care 1).

Note: If you choose to work during Period of Care 4: 1900-2000, the Patient List screen is skipped since you are not able to visit patients or administer medications during the shift. Instead, you are taken directly to the Nurses' Station, where the records of all the patients on the floor are available for your review.

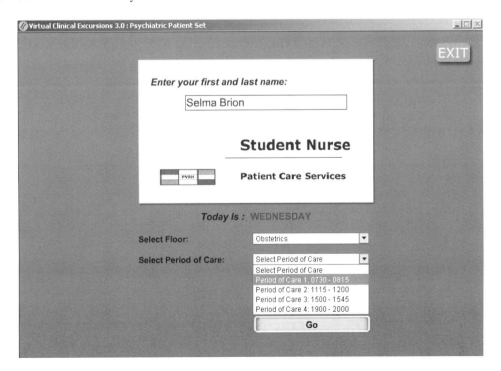

Copyright © 2011, 2007 by Mosby, Inc., an affiliate of Elsevier Inc. All rights reserved.

PATIENT LIST

OBSTETRICS UNIT

Dorothy Grant (Room 201)
30-week intrauterine pregnancy—A 25-year-old multipara Caucasian female admitted with abdominal trauma following a domestic violence incident. Her complications include preterm labor and extensive social issues such as acquiring safe housing for her family upon discharge.

Kelly Brady (Room 203)
26-week intrauterine pregnancy—A 35-year-old primigravida Caucasian female urgently admitted for progressive symptoms of preeclampsia. A history of inadequate coping with major life stressors leave her at risk for a recurrence of depression as she faces a diagnosis of HELLP syndrome and the delivery of a severely premature infant.

Laura Wilson (Room 206)
37-week intrauterine pregnancy—An 18-year-old primigravida Caucasian female urgently admitted after being found unconscious. Her complications include HIV-positive status and chronic polysubstance abuse. Unrealistic expectations of parenthood and living with a chronic illness, combined with strained family relations, prompt comprehensive social and psychiatric evaluations initiated on the day of simulation.

PEDIATRIC UNIT

Tiffany Sheldon (Room 305)
Anorexia nervosa—A 14-year-old Caucasian female admitted for dehydration, electrolyte imbalance, and malnutrition following a syncope episode at home. This patient has a history of eating disorders that have required multiple hospital admissions and have strained family dynamics between mother and daughter.

MEDICAL-SURGICAL UNIT

Harry George (Room 401)
Osteomyelitis—A 54-year-old Caucasian male admitted from a homeless shelter with an infected leg. He has complications of type 2 diabetes mellitus, alcohol abuse, nicotine addiction, poor pain control, and complex psychosocial issues.

Jacquline Catanazaro (Room 402)
Asthma—A 45-year-old Caucasian female admitted with an acute asthma exacerbation and suspected pneumonia. She has complications of chronic schizophrenia, noncompliance with medication therapy, obesity, and herniated disk.

SKILLED NURSING UNIT

Kathryn Doyle (Room 503)
Rehabilitation post left hip replacement—A 79-year-old Caucasian female admitted following a complicated recovery from an ORIF. She is experiencing symptoms of malnutrition and depression due to unstable family dynamics, placing her at risk for elder abuse.

Carlos Reyes (Room 504)
Rehabilitation status post myocardial infarction—An 81-year-old Hispanic male admitted for evaluation of the need for long-term care following an acute care hospital stay. Recent cognitive changes and a diagnosis of anxiety disorder contribute to stressful family dynamics and caregiver strain.

■ HOW TO SELECT A PATIENT

- You can choose one or more patients to work with from the Patient List by checking the box to the left of the patient name(s). For this quick tour, select Dorothy Grant. (In order to receive a scorecard for a patient, the patient must be selected before proceeding to the Nurses' Station.)
- Click on **Get Report** to the right of the medical records number (MRN) to view a summary of the patient's care during the 12-hour period before your arrival on the unit.
- After reviewing the report, click on **Go to Nurses' Station** in the right lower corner to begin your care. (*Note:* If you have been assigned to care for multiple patients, you can click on **Return to Patient List** to select and review the report for each additional patient before going to the Nurses' Station.)

Note: Even though the Patient List is initially skipped when you sign in to work for Period of Care 4, you can still access this screen if you wish to review the shift report for any of the patients. To do so, simply click on **Patient List** near the top left corner of the Nurses' Station (or click on the clipboard to the left of the Kardex). Then click on **Get Report** for the patient(s) whose care you are reviewing. This may be done during any period of care.

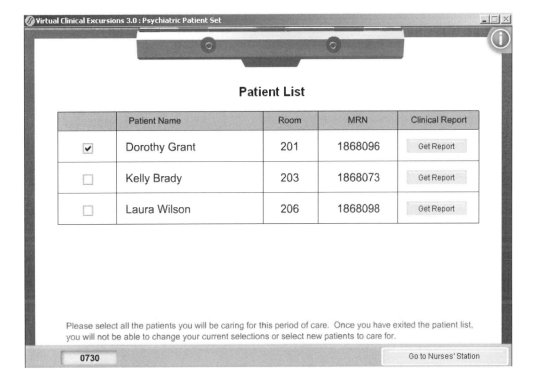

12 GETTING STARTED

■ HOW TO FIND A PATIENT'S RECORDS

NURSES' STATION

Within the Nurses' Station, you will see:

1. A clipboard that contains the patient list for that floor.
2. A chart rack with patient charts labeled by room number, a notebook labeled Kardex, and a notebook labeled MAR (Medication Administration Record).
3. A desktop computer with access to the Electronic Patient Record (EPR).
4. A tool bar across the top of the screen that can also be used to access the Patient List, EPR, Chart, MAR, and Kardex. This tool bar is also accessible from each patient's room.
5. A Drug Guide containing information about the medications you are able to administer to your patients.
6. A tool bar across the bottom of the screen that can be used to access the Floor Map, patient rooms, Medication Room, and Drug Guide.

As you run your cursor over an item, it will be highlighted. To select, simply click on the item. As you use these resources, you will always be able to return to the Nurses' Station by clicking on the **Return to Nurses' Station** bar located in the right lower corner of your screen.

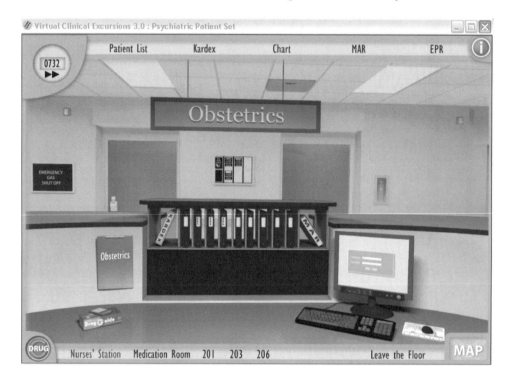

Copyright © 2011, 2007 by Mosby, Inc., an affiliate of Elsevier Inc. All rights reserved.

MEDICATION ADMINISTRATION RECORD (MAR)

The MAR icon located on the tool bar at the top of your screen accesses current 24-hour medications for each patient. Click on the icon and the MAR will open. (*Note:* You can also access the MAR by clicking on the MAR notebook on the far right side of the book rack in the center of the screen.) Within the MAR, tabs on the right side of the screen allow you to select patients by room number. Be careful to make sure you select the correct tab number for *your* patient rather than simply reading the first record that appears after the MAR opens. Each MAR sheet lists the following:

- Medications
- Route and dosage of each medication
- Times of administration of each medication

Note: The MAR changes each day. Expired MARs are stored in the patients' charts.

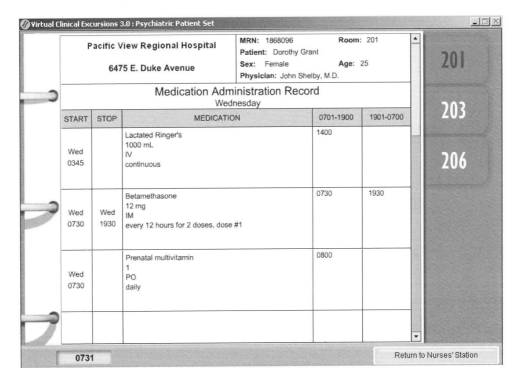

14 GETTING STARTED

CHARTS

To access patient charts, either click on the **Chart** icon at the top of your screen or anywhere within the chart rack in the center of the Nurses' Station screen. When the close-up view appears, the individual charts are labeled by room number. To open a chart, click on the room number of the patient whose chart you wish to review. The patient's name and allergies will appear on the left side of the screen, along with a list of tabs on the right side of the screen, allowing you to view the following data:

- Allergies
- Physician's Orders
- Physician's Notes
- Nurse's Notes
- Laboratory Reports
- Diagnostic Reports
- Surgical Reports
- Consultations
- Patient Education
- History and Physical
- Nursing Admission
- Expired MARs
- Consents
- Mental Health
- Admissions
- Emergency Department

Information appears in real time. The entries are in reverse chronologic order, so use the down arrow at the right side of each chart page to scroll down to view previous entries. Flip from tab to tab to view multiple data fields or click on **Return to Nurses' Station** in the lower right corner of the screen to exit the chart.

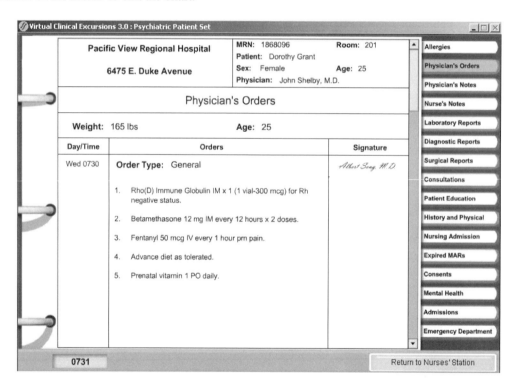

Copyright © 2011, 2007 by Mosby, Inc., an affiliate of Elsevier Inc. All rights reserved.

Electronic Patient Record (EPR)

The EPR can be accessed from the computer in the Nurses' Station or from the EPR icon located in the tool bar at the top of your screen. To access a patient's EPR:
- Click on either the computer screen or the **EPR** icon.
- Your username and password are automatically filled in.
- Click on **Login** to enter the EPR.
- *Note:* Like the MAR, the EPR is arranged numerically. Thus when you enter, you are initially shown the records of the patient in the lowest room number on the floor. To view the correct data for *your* patient, remember to select the correct room number, using the drop-down menu for the Patient field at the top left corner of the screen.

The EPR used in Pacific View Regional Hospital represents a composite of commercial versions being used in hospitals. You can access the EPR:
- to review existing data for a patient (by room number).
- to enter data you collect while working with a patient.

The EPR is updated daily, so no matter what day or part of a shift you are working, there will be a current EPR with the patient's data from the past days of the current hospital stay. This type of simulated EPR allows you to examine how data for different attributes have changed over time, as well as to examine data for all of a patient's attributes at a particular time. The EPR is fully functional (as it is in a real-life hospital). You can enter such data as blood pressure, breath sounds, and certain treatments. The EPR will not, however, allow you to enter data for a previous time period. Use the arrows at the bottom of the screen to move forward and backward in time.

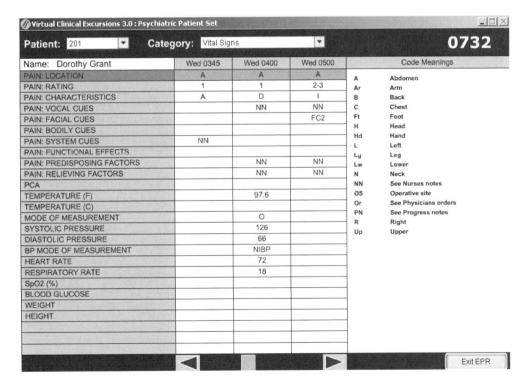

At the top of the EPR screen, you can choose patients by their room numbers. In addition, you have access to 17 different categories of patient data. To change patients or data categories, click the down arrow to the right of the room number or category.

The categories of patient data in the EPR are as follows:

- Vital Signs
- Respiratory
- Cardiovascular
- Neurologic
- Gastrointestinal
- Excretory
- Musculoskeletal
- Integumentary
- Reproductive
- Psychosocial
- Wounds and Drains
- Activity
- Hygiene and Comfort
- Safety
- Nutrition
- IV
- Intake and Output

Remember, each hospital selects its own codes. The codes used in the EPR at Pacific View Regional Hospital may be different from ones you have seen in your clinical rotations. Take some time to acquaint yourself with the codes. Within the Vital Signs category, click on any item in the left column (e.g., Pain: Characteristics). In the far-right column, you will see a list of code meanings for the possible findings and/or descriptors for that assessment area.

You will use the codes to record the data you collect as you work with patients. Click on the box in the last time column to the right of any item and wait for the code meanings applicable to that entry to appear. Select the appropriate code to describe your assessment findings and type it in the box. (*Note:* If no cursor appears within the box, click on the box again until the blue shading disappears and the blinking cursor appears.) Once the data are typed in this box, they are entered into the patient's record for this period of care only.

To leave the EPR, click on **Exit EPR** in the bottom right corner of the screen.

■ VISITING A PATIENT

From the Nurses' Station, click on the room number of the patient you wish to visit (in the tool bar at the bottom of your screen). Once you are inside the room, you will see a still photo of your patient in the top left corner. To verify that this is the correct patient, click on the **Check Armband** icon to the right of the photo. The patient's identification data will appear. If you click on **Check Allergies** (the next icon to the right), a list of the patient's allergies (if any) will replace the photo.

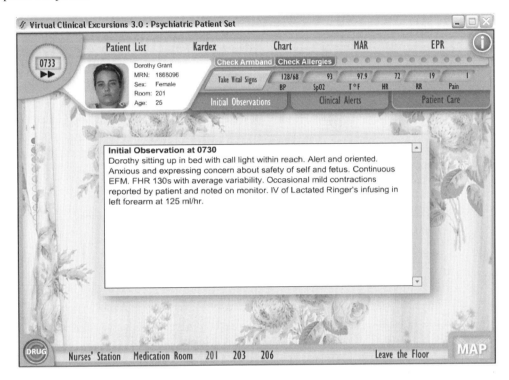

Also located in the patient's room are multiple icons you can use to assess the patient or the patient's medications. A virtual clock is provided in the upper left corner of the room to monitor your progress in real time. (*Note:* The fast forward icon within the virtual clock will advance the time by 2-minute intervals when clicked.)

- The tool bar across the top of the screen allows you to check the **Patient List**, access the **EPR** to check or enter data, and view the patient's **Chart**, **MAR**, or **Kardex**.

- The **Take Vital Signs** icon allows you to measure the patient's up-to-the-minute blood pressure, oxygen saturation, temperature, heart rate, respiratory rate, and pain level.

- Each time you enter a patient's room, you are given an Initial Observation report to review (in the text box under the patient's photo). These notes are provided to give you a "look" at the patient as if you had just stepped into the room. You can also click on the **Initial Observations** icon to return to this box from other views within the patient's room. To the right of this icon is **Clinical Alerts**, a resource that allows you to make decisions about priority medication interventions based on emerging data collected in real time. Check this screen throughout your period of care to avoid missing critical information related to recently ordered or STAT medications.

- Clicking on **Patient Care** opens up three specific learning environments within the patient room: **Physical Assessment**, **Nurse-Client Interactions**, and **Medication Administration**.

- To perform a **Physical Assessment**, choose a body area (such as **Head & Neck**) from the column of yellow buttons. This activates a list of system subcategories for that body area (e.g., see **Sensory**, **Neurologic**, etc. in the green boxes). After you select the system you

Copyright © 2011, 2007 by Mosby, Inc., an affiliate of Elsevier Inc. All rights reserved.

18 GETTING STARTED

wish to evaluate, a brief description of the assessment findings will appear in a box to the right. A still photo provides a "snapshot" of how an assessment of this area might be done or what the finding might look like. For every body area, you can also click on **Equipment** on the right side of the screen.

- To the right of the Physical Assessment icon is **Nurse-Client Interactions**. Clicking on this icon will reveal the times and titles of any videos available for viewing. (*Note:* If the video you wish to see is not listed, this means you have not yet reached the correct virtual time to view that video. Check the virtual clock; you may return to access the video once its designated time has occurred—as long as you do so within the same period of care. Or you can click on the fast-forward icon within the virtual clock to advance the time by 2-minute intervals. You will then need to click again on **Patient Care** and **Nurse-Client Interactions** to refresh the screen.) To view a listed video, click on the white arrow to the right of the video title. Use the control buttons below the video to start, stop, pause, rewind, or fast-forward the action or to mute the sound.

- **Medication Administration** is the pathway that allows you to review and administer medications to a patient after you have prepared them in the Medication Room. This process is addressed further in the *How to Prepare Medications* section (pages 19-20) and in *Medications* (pages 26-30). For additional hands-on practice, see *Reducing Medication Errors* (pages 37-41).

■ HOW TO QUIT, CHANGE PATIENTS, CHANGE FLOORS, OR CHANGE PERIODS OF CARE

How to Quit: From most screens, you may click the **Leave the Floor** icon on the bottom tool bar to the right of the patient room numbers. (*Note:* From some screens, you will first need to click an **Exit** button or **Return to Nurses' Station** before clicking **Leave the Floor**.) When the Floor Menu appears, click **Exit** to leave the program.

How to Change Patients, Floors, or Periods of Care: To change patients, simply click on the new patient's room number. (You cannot receive a scorecard for a new patient, however, unless you have already selected that patient on the Patient List screen.) To change to a new period of care, to change floors, or to restart the virtual clock, click on **Leave the Floor** and then on **Restart the Program**.

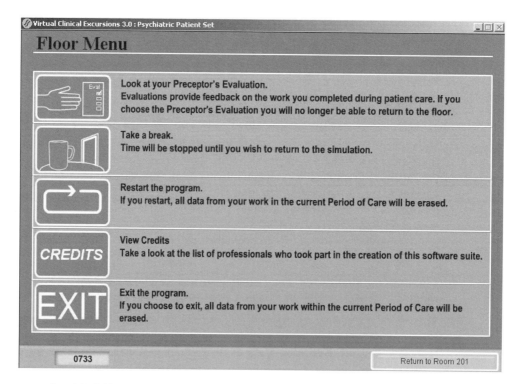

Copyright © 2011, 2007 by Mosby, Inc., an affiliate of Elsevier Inc. All rights reserved.

A QUICK TOUR   19

■ HOW TO PREPARE MEDICATIONS

From the Nurses' Station or the patient's room, you can access the Medication Room by clicking on the icon in the tool bar at the bottom of your screen to the left of the patient room numbers.

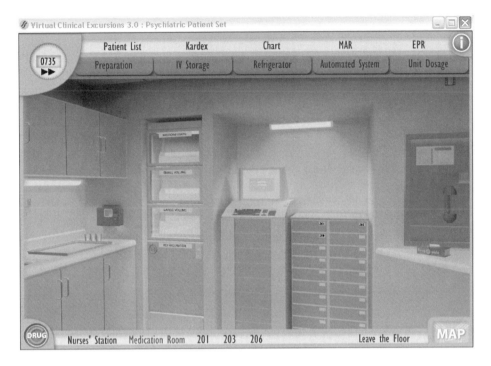

In the Medication Room you have access to the following (from left to right):

- A preparation area is located on the counter under the cabinets. To begin the medication preparation process, click on the tray on the counter or click on the **Preparation** icon at the top of the screen. The next screen leads you through a specific sequence (called the Preparation Wizard) to prepare medications one at a time for administration to a patient. However, no medication has been selected at this time. We will do this while working with a patient in *A Detailed Tour*. To exit this screen, click on **View Medication Room**.

- To the right of the cabinets (and above the refrigerator), IV storage bins are provided. Click on the bins themselves or on the **IV Storage** icon at the top of the screen. The bins are labeled **Microinfusion**, **Small Volume**, and **Large Volume**. Click on an individual bin to see a list of its contents. If you needed to prepare an IV medication at this time, you could click on the medication and its label would appear to the right under the patient's name. (*Note:* You can **Open** and **Close** any medication label by clicking the appropriate icon.) Next, you would click **Put Medication on Tray**. If you ever change your mind or decide that you have put the incorrect medication on the tray, you can reverse your actions by highlighting the medication on the tray and then clicking **Put Medication in Bin**. Click **Close Bin** in the right bottom corner to exit. **View Medication Room** brings you back to a full view of the entire room.

- A refrigerator is located under the IV storage bins to hold any medications that must be stored below room temperature. Click on the refrigerator door or on the **Refrigerator** icon at the top of the screen. Then click on the close-up view of the door to access the medications. When you are finished, click **Close Door** and then **View Medication Room**.

Copyright © 2011, 2007 by Mosby, Inc., an affiliate of Elsevier Inc. All rights reserved.

20 GETTING STARTED

- To prepare controlled substances, click the **Automated System** icon at the top of the screen or click the computer monitor located to the right of the IV storage bins. A login screen will appear; your name and password are automatically filled in. Click **Login**. Select the patient for whom you wish to access medications; then select the correct medication drawer to open (they are stored alphabetically). Click **Open Drawer**, highlight the proper medication, and choose **Put Medication on Tray**. When you are finished, click **Close Drawer** and then **View Medication Room**.

- Next to the Automated System is a set of drawers identified by patient room number. To access these, click on the drawers or on the **Unit Dosage** icon at the top of the screen. This provides a close-up view of the drawers. To open a drawer, click on the room number of the patient you are working with. Next, click on the medication you would like to prepare for the patient, and a label will appear, listing the medication strength, units, and dosage per unit. To exit, click **Close Drawer**; then click **View Medication Room**.

At any time, you can learn about a medication you wish to prepare for a patient by clicking on the **Drug** icon in the bottom left corner of the medication room screen or by clicking the **Drug Guide** book on the counter to the right of the unit dosage drawers. The **Drug Guide** provides information about the medications commonly included in nursing drug handbooks. Nutritional supplements and maintenance intravenous fluid preparations are not included. Highlight a medication in the alphabetical list; relevant information about the drug will appear in the screen below. To exit, click **Return to Medication Room**.

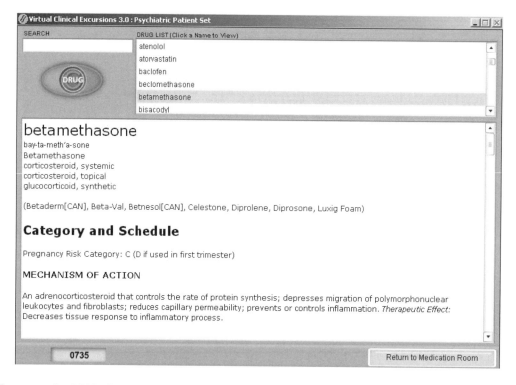

To access the MAR from the Medication Room and to review the medications ordered for a patient, click on the **MAR** icon located in the tool bar at the top of your screen and then click on the correct tab for your patient's room number. You may also click the **Review MAR** icon in the tool bar at the bottom of your screen from inside each medication storage area.

After you have chosen and prepared medications, go to the patient's room to administer them by clicking on the room number in the bottom tool bar. Inside the patient's room, click **Patient Care** and then **Medication Administration** and follow the proper administration sequence.

A QUICK TOUR

■ PRECEPTOR'S EVALUATIONS

When you have finished a session, click on **Leave the Floor** to go to the Floor Menu. At this point, you can click on the top icon (**Look at Your Preceptor's Evaluation**) to receive a scorecard that provides feedback on the work you completed during patient care.

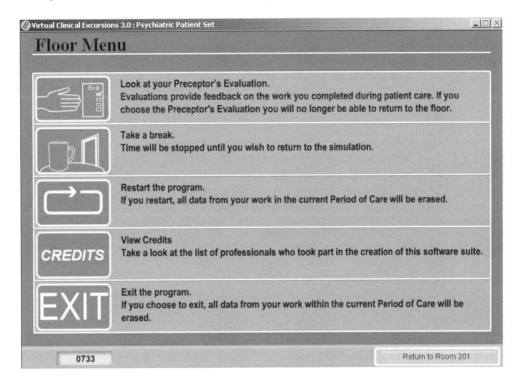

Evaluations are available for each patient you selected when you signed in for the current period of care. Click on the **Medication Scorecard** icon to see an example.

22 Getting Started

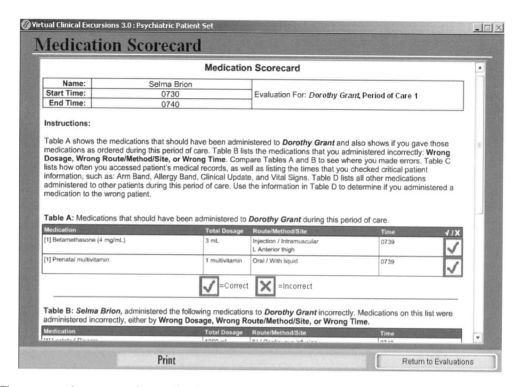

The scorecard compares the medications you administered to a patient during a period of care with what should have been administered. Table A lists the correct medications. Table B lists any medications that were administered incorrectly.

Remember, not every medication listed on the MAR should necessarily be given. For example, a patient might have an allergy to a drug that was ordered, or a medication might have been improperly transcribed to the MAR. Predetermined medication "errors" embedded within the program challenge you to exercise critical thinking skills and professional judgment when deciding to administer a medication, just as you would in a real hospital. Use all your available resources, such as the patient's chart and the MAR, to make your decision.

Table C lists the resources that were available to assist you in medication administration. It also documents whether and when you accessed these resources. For example, did you check the patient armband or perform a check of vital signs? If so, when?

You can click **Print** to get a copy of this report if needed. When you have finished reviewing the scorecard, click **Return to Evaluations** and then **Return to Menu**.

A QUICK TOUR   23

■ **FLOOR MAP**

To get a general sense of your location within the hospital, you can click on the **Map** icon found in the lower right corner of most of the screens in the *Virtual Clinical Excursions—Psychiatric* program. (*Note:* If you are following this quick tour step by step, you will need to **Restart the Program** from the Floor Menu, sign in again, and go to the Nurses' Station to access the map.) When you click the **Map** icon, a floor map appears, showing the layout of the floor you are currently on, as well as a directory of the patients and services on that floor. As you move your cursor over the directory list, the location of each room is highlighted on the map (and vice versa). The floor map can be accessed from the Nurses' Station, Medication Room, and each patient's room.

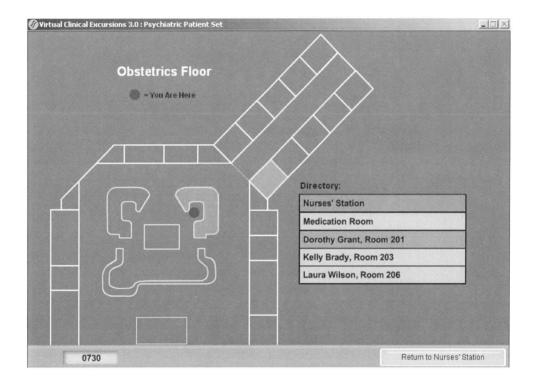

A DETAILED TOUR

If you wish to more thoroughly understand the capabilities of *Virtual Clinical Excursions—Psychiatric*, take a detailed tour by completing the following section. During this tour, we will work with a specific patient to introduce you to all the different components and learning opportunities available within the software.

■ WORKING WITH A PATIENT

Sign in and select the Obstetrics Floor for Period of Care 1 (0730-0815). From the Patient List, select Dorothy Grant in Room 201; however, do not go to the Nurses' Station yet.

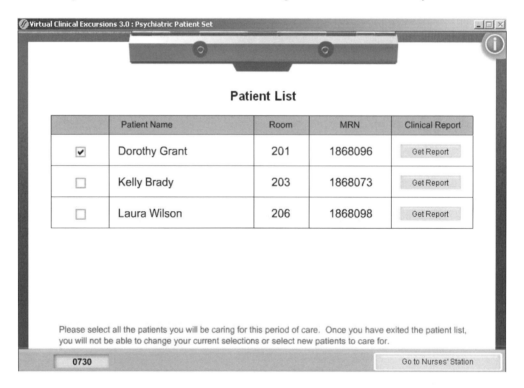

■ REPORT

In hospitals, when one shift ends and another begins, the outgoing nurse who attended a patient will give a verbal and sometimes a written summary of that patient's condition to the incoming nurse who will assume care for the patient. This summary is called a report and is an important source of data to provide an overview of a patient. Your first task is to get the clinical report on Dorothy Grant. To do this, click **Get Report** in the far right column in this patient's row. From a brief review of this summary, identify the problems and areas of concern that you will need to address for this patient.

When you have finished noting any areas of concern, click on **Go to Nurses' Station**.

■ CHARTS

You can access Dorothy Grant's chart from the Nurses' Station or from the patient's room (201). From the Nurses' Station, click on the chart rack or on the **Chart** icon in the tool bar at the top of your screen. Next, click on the chart labeled **201** to open the medical record for Dorothy Grant. Click on the **Emergency Department** tab to view a record of why this patient was admitted.

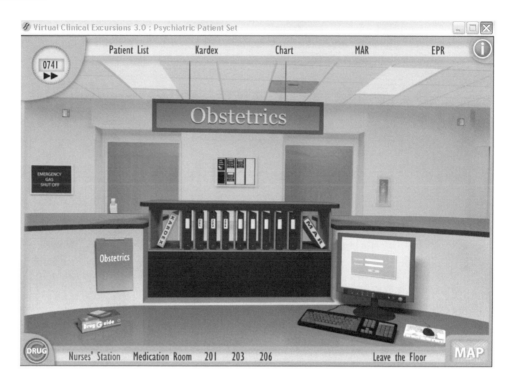

How many days has Dorothy Grant been in the hospital?

What tests were done upon her arrival in the Emergency Department and why?

What was her reason for admission?

You should also click on **Diagnostic Reports** to learn what additional tests or procedures were performed and when. Finally, review the **Nursing Admission** and **History and Physical** to learn about the health history of this patient. When you are done reviewing the chart, click **Return to Nurses' Station**.

26 GETTING STARTED

■ MEDICATIONS

Open the Medication Administration Record (MAR) by clicking on the **MAR** icon in the tool bar at the top of your screen. *Remember:* The MAR automatically opens to the first occupied room number on the floor—which is not necessarily your patient's room number! Since you need to access Dorothy Grant's MAR, click on tab **201** (her room number). Always make sure you are giving the *Right Drug to the Right Patient!*

Examine the list of medications ordered for Dorothy Grant. In the table below, list the medications that need to be given during this period of care (0730-0815). For each medication, note the dosage, route, and time to be given.

Time	Medication	Dosage	Route

Click on **Return to Nurses' Station**. Next, click on **201** on the bottom tool bar and then verify that you are indeed in Dorothy Grant's room. Select **Clinical Alerts** (the icon to the right of Initial Observations) to check for any emerging data that might affect your medication administration priorities. Next, go to the patient's chart (click on the **Chart** icon; then click on **201**). When the chart opens, select the **Physician's Orders** tab.

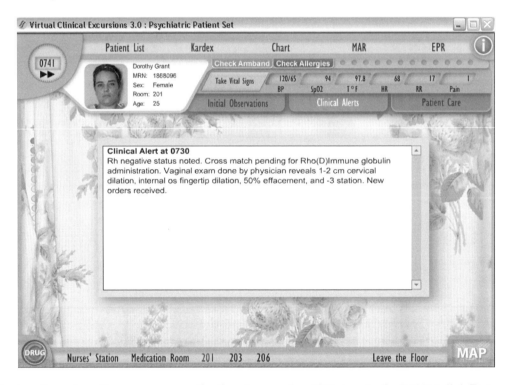

Review the orders. Have any new medications been ordered? Return to the MAR (click **Return to Room 201**; then click **MAR**). Verify that any new medications have been correctly transcribed to the MAR. Mistakes are sometimes made in the transcription process in the hospital setting, and it is sound practice to double-check any new order.

Copyright © 2011, 2007 by Mosby, Inc., an affiliate of Elsevier Inc. All rights reserved.

A Detailed Tour

Are there any patient assessments you will need to perform before administering these medications? If so, return to Room 201 and click on **Patient Care** and then **Physical Assessment** to complete those assessments before proceeding.

Now click on the **Medication Room** icon in the tool bar at the bottom of your screen to locate and prepare the medications for Dorothy Grant.

In the Medication Room, you must access the medications for Dorothy Grant from the specific dispensing system in which each medication is stored. Locate each medication that needs to be given in this time period and click on **Put Medication on Tray** as appropriate. (*Hint:* Look in **Unit Dosage** drawer first.) When you are finished, click on **Close Drawer** and then on **View Medication Room**. Now click on the medication tray on the counter on the left side of the medication room screen to begin preparing the medications you have selected. (*Remember:* You can also click **Preparation** in the tool bar at the top of the screen.)

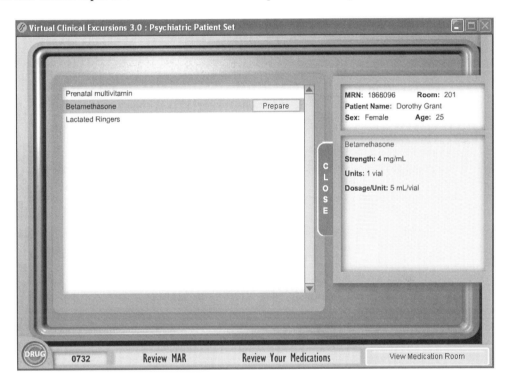

In the preparation area, you should see a list of the medications you put on the tray in the previous steps. Click on the first medication and then click **Prepare**. Follow the onscreen instructions of the Preparation Wizard, providing any data requested. As an example, let's follow the preparation process for betamethasone, one of the medications due to be administered to Dorothy Grant during this period of care. To begin, click to select **Betamethasone**; then click **Prepare**. Now work through the Preparation Wizard sequence as detailed below:

> Amount of medication in the ampule: 5 mL.
> Enter the amount of medication you will draw up into a syringe: **3 mL**.
> Click **Next**.
> Select the patient to receive the medication: **Room 201, Dorothy Grant**.
> Click **Finish**.
> Click **Return to Medication Room**.

Copyright © 2011, 2007 by Mosby, Inc., an affiliate of Elsevier Inc. All rights reserved.

28 GETTING STARTED

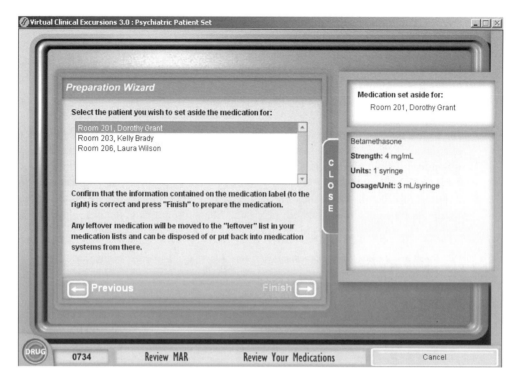

Follow this same basic process for the other medications due to be administered to Dorothy Grant during this period of care. (*Hint:* Look in **IV Storage** and **Automated System**.)

PREPARATION WIZARD EXCEPTIONS

- Some medications in *Virtual Clinical Excursions—Psychiatric* are prepared by the pharmacy (e.g., IV antibiotics) and taken to the patient room as a whole. This is common practice in most hospitals.
- Blood products are not administered by students through the *Virtual Clinical Excursions—Psychiatric* simulations since blood administration follows specific protocols not covered in this program.
- The *Virtual Clinical Excursions—Psychiatric* simulations do not allow for mixing more than one type of medication, such as regular and Lente insulins, in the same syringe. In the clinical setting, when multiple types of insulin are ordered for a patient, the regular insulin is drawn up first, followed by the longer-acting insulin. Insulin is always administered in a special unit-marked syringe.

Now return to Room 201 (click on **201** on the bottom tool bar) to administer Dorothy Grant's medications.

At any time during the medication administration process, you can perform a further review of systems, take vital signs, check information contained within the chart, or verify patient identity and allergies. Inside Dorothy Grant's room, click **Take Vital Signs**. (*Note:* These findings change over time to reflect the temporal changes you would find in a patient similar to Dorothy Grant.)

A DETAILED TOUR

When you have gathered all the data you need, click on **Patient Care** and then select **Medication Administration**. Any medications you prepared in the previous steps should be listed on the left side of your screen. Let's continue the administration process with the betamethasone ordered for Dorothy Grant. Click to highlight **Betamethasone** in the list of medications. Next, click on the down arrow to the right of **Select** and choose **Administer** from the drop-down menu. This will activate the Administration Wizard. Complete the Wizard sequence as follows:

- Route: **Injection**
- Method: **Intramuscular**
- Site: **Any** (choose one)
- Click **Administer to Patient** arrow.
- Would you like to document this administration in the MAR? **Yes**
- Click **Finish** arrow.

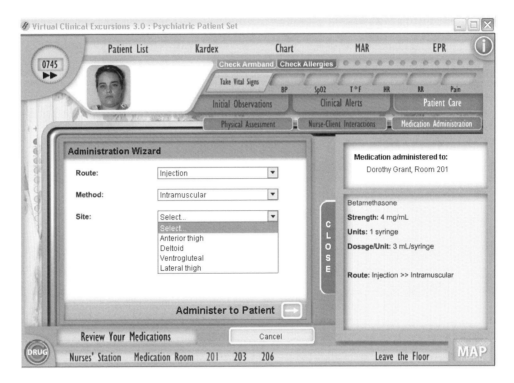

Your selections are recorded by a tracking system and evaluated on a Medication Scorecard stored under Preceptor's Evaluations. This scorecard can be viewed, printed, and given to your instructor. To access the Preceptor's Evaluations, click on **Leave the Floor**. When the Floor Menu appears, select **Look at Your Preceptor's Evaluation**. Then click on **Medication Scorecard** inside the box with Dorothy Grant's name (see example on the following page).

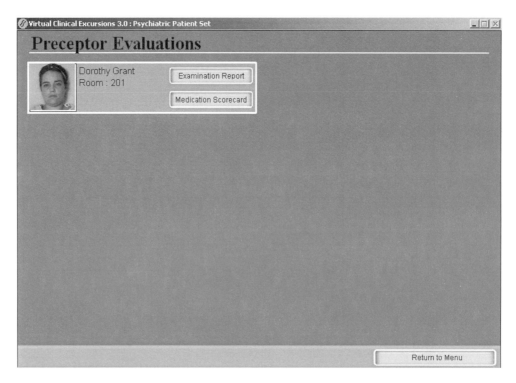

■ MEDICATION SCORECARD

- First, review Table A. Was betamethasone given correctly? Did you give the other medications as ordered?
- Table B shows you which (if any) medications you gave incorrectly.
- Table C addresses the resources used for Dorothy Grant. Did you access the patient's chart, MAR, EPR, or Kardex as needed to make safe medication administration decisions?
- Did you check the patient's armband to verify her identity? Did you check whether your patient had any known allergies to medications? Were vital signs taken?

When you have finished reviewing the scorecard, click **Return to Evaluations** and then **Return to Menu**.

■ VITAL SIGNS

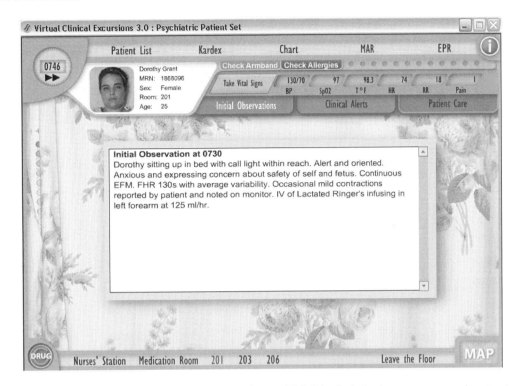

Vital signs, often considered the traditional "signs of life," include body temperature, heart rate, respiratory rate, blood pressure, oxygen saturation of the blood, and pain level.

Inside Dorothy Grant's room, click **Take Vital Signs**. (*Note:* If you are following this detailed tour step by step, you will need to **Restart the Program** from the Floor Menu, sign in again for Period of Care 1, and navigate to Room 201.) Collect vital signs for this patient and record them below. Note the time at which you collected each of these data. (*Remember:* You can take vital signs at any time. The data change over time to reflect the temporal changes you would find in a patient similar to Dorothy Grant.)

Vital Signs	Findings/Time
Blood pressure	
O_2 saturation	
Temperature	
Heart rate	
Respiratory rate	
Pain rating	

Copyright © 2011, 2007 by Mosby, Inc., an affiliate of Elsevier Inc. All rights reserved.

32 GETTING STARTED

After you are done, click on the **EPR** icon located in the tool bar at the top of the screen. Your username and password are automatically provided. Click on **Login** to enter the EPR. To access Dorothy Grant's records, click on the down arrow next to Patient and choose her room number, **201**. Select **Vital Signs** as the category. Next, in the empty time column on the far right, record the vital signs data you just collected in Dorothy Grant's room. (*Note:* If you need help with this process, see page 16.) Now compare these findings with the data you collected earlier for this patient's vital signs. Use these earlier findings to establish a baseline for each of the vital signs.

    a. Are any of the data you collected significantly different from the baseline for a particular vital sign?

       Circle One: Yes   No

    b. If "Yes," which data are different?

■ **PHYSICAL ASSESSMENT**

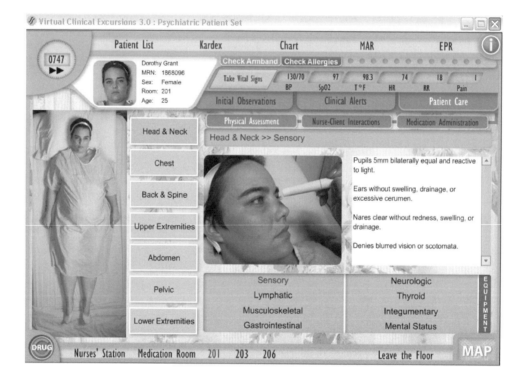

After you have finished examining the EPR for vital signs, click **Exit EPR** to return to Room 201. Click **Patient Care** and then **Physical Assessment**. Think about the information you received in the report at the beginning of this shift, as well as what you may have learned about this patient from the chart. Based on this, what area(s) of examination should you pay most attention to at this time? Is there any equipment you should be monitoring? Conduct a physical assessment of the body areas and systems that you consider priorities for Dorothy Grant. For example, select **Head & Neck**; then click on and assess **Sensory** and **Lymphatic**. Complete any other assessment(s) you think are necessary at this time. In the following table, record the data you collected during this examination.

Area of Examination	**Findings**
Head & Neck Sensory	
Head & Neck Lymphatic	

After you have finished collecting these data, return to the EPR. Compare the data that were already in the record with those you just collected.

    a. Are any of the data you collected significantly different from the baselines for this patient?

        Circle One: Yes   No

    b. If "Yes," which data are different?

■ NURSE-CLIENT INTERACTIONS

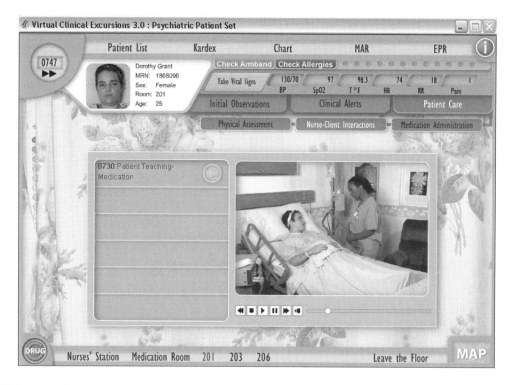

Click on **Patient Care** from inside Dorothy Grant's room (201). Now click on **Nurse-Client Interactions** to access a short video titled **Patient Teaching—Medication**, which is available for viewing at or after 0730 (based on the virtual clock in the upper left corner of your screen; see *Note* below). To begin the video, click on the white arrow next to its title. You will observe a nurse communicating with Dorothy Grant. There are many variations of nursing practice, some exemplifying "best" practice and some not. Note whether the nurse in this interaction displays professional behavior and compassionate care. Are her words congruent with what is going on with the patient? Does this interaction "feel right" to you? If not, how would you handle this situation differently? Explain.

Note: If the video you wish to view is not listed, this means you have not yet reached the correct virtual time to view that video. Check the virtual clock; you may return to access the video once its designated time has occurred—as long as you do so within the same period of care. Or you can click on the fast-forward icon within the virtual clock to advance the time by 2-minute intervals. You will then need to click again on **Patient Care** and **Nurse-Client Interactions** to refresh the screen.

At least one Nurse-Client Interactions video is available during each period of care. Viewing these videos can help you learn more about what is occurring with a patient at a certain time and also prompt you to discern between nurse communications that are ideal and those that need improvement. Compassionate care and the ability to communicate clearly are essential components of delivering quality nursing care, and it is during your clinical time that you will begin to refine these skills.

■ COLLECTING AND EVALUATING DATA

Each of the activities you perform in the Patient Care environment generates a significant amount of assessment data. Remember that after you collect data, you can record your findings in the EPR. You can also review the EPR, patient's chart, videos, and MAR at any time. You will get plenty of practice collecting and then evaluating data in context of the patient's course.

Now, here's an important question for you:

> Did the previous sequence of exercises provide the most efficient way to assess Dorothy Grant?

For example, you went to the patient's room to get vital signs, then back to the EPR to enter data and compare your findings with extant data. Next, you went back to the patient's room to do a physical examination, then again back to the EPR to enter and review data. If this back-and-forth process of data collection and recording seemed inefficient, remember the following:

- Plan all of your nursing activities to maximize efficiency, while at the same time optimizing the quality of patient care. (Think about what data you might need before performing certain tasks. For example, do you need to check a heart rate before administering a cardiac medication or check an IV site before starting an infusion?)

- You collect a tremendous amount of data when you work with a patient. Very few people can accurately remember all these data for more than a few minutes. Develop efficient assessment skills, and record data as soon as possible after collecting them.

- Assessment data are only the starting point for the nursing process.

Make a clear distinction between these first exercises and how you actually provide nursing care. These initial exercises were designed to involve you actively in the use of different software components. This workbook focuses on sensible practices for implementing the nursing process in ways that ensure the highest-quality care of patients.

Most important, remember that a human being changes through time, and that these changes include both the physical and psychosocial facets of a person as a living organism. Think about this for a moment. Some patients may change physically in a very short time (a patient with emerging myocardial infarction) or more slowly (a patient with a chronic illness). Patients' overall physical and psychosocial conditions may improve or deteriorate. They may have effective coping skills and familial support, or they may feel alone and full of despair. In fact, each individual is a complex mix of physical and psychosocial elements, and at least some of these elements usually change through time.

Thus it is crucial that you *DO NOT* think of the nursing process as a simple one-time, five-step procedure consisting of assessment, nursing diagnosis, planning, implementation, and evaluation. Rather, the nursing process should be utilized as a creative and systematic approach to delivering nursing care. Furthermore, because all living organisms are constantly changing, we must apply the nursing process over and over. Each time we follow the nursing process for an individual patient, we refine our understanding of that patient's physical and psychosocial conditions based on collection and analysis of many different types of data. *Virtual Clinical Excursions—Psychiatric* will help you develop both the creativity and the systematic approach needed to become a nurse who is equipped to deliver the highest-quality care to all patients.

REDUCING MEDICATION ERRORS

Earlier in this detailed tour, you learned the basic steps of medication preparation and administration. The following simulations will allow you to practice those skills further—with an increased emphasis on reducing medication errors by using the Medication Scorecard to evaluate your work.

Sign in to work on the Obstetrics Floor at Pacific View Regional Hospital for Period of Care 1. (*Note:* If you are already working with another patient or during another period of care, click on **Leave the Floor** and then **Restart the Program**; then sign in.)

From the Patient List, select Dorothy Grant. Then click on **Go to Nurses' Station**. Complete the following steps to prepare and administer medications to Dorothy Grant.

- Click on **Medication Room** on the toolbar at the bottom of your screen.
- Click on **MAR** and then on tab **201** to determine medications that have been ordered for Dorothy Grant. (*Note:* You may click on **Review MAR** at any time to verify the correct medication orders. Always remember to check the patient name on the MAR to make sure you have the correct patient's record—you must click on the correct room number tab within the MAR.) Click on **Return to Medication Room** after reviewing the correct MAR.
- Click on **Unit Dosage** (or on the Unit Dosage cabinet); from the close-up view, click on drawer **201**.
- Select the medications you would like to administer. After each selection, click **Put Medication on Tray**. When you are finished selecting medications, click **Close Drawer** and then **View Medication Room**.
- Click on **Automated System** (or on the Automated System unit itself). Click **Login**.
- On the next screen, specify the correct patient and drawer location.
- Select the medication you would like to administer and click **Put Medication on Tray**. Repeat this process if you wish to administer other medications from the Automated System.
- When you are finished, click **Close Drawer** and **View Medication Room**.
- From the Medication Room, click **Preparation** (or on the preparation tray).
- From the list of medications on your tray, highlight the correct medication to administer and click **Prepare**.
- This activates the Preparation Wizard. Supply any requested information; then click **Next**.
- Now select the correct patient to receive this medication and click **Finish**.
- Repeat the previous three steps until all medications that you want to administer are prepared.
- You can click **Review Your Medications** and then **Return to Medication Room** when ready. Once you are back in the Medication Room, go directly to Dorothy Grant's room by clicking on **201** at the bottom of the screen.
- Inside the patient's room, administer the medication, utilizing the six rights of medication administration. After you have collected the appropriate assessment data and are ready for administration, click **Patient Care** and then **Medication Administration**. Verify that the correct patient and medication(s) appear in the left-hand window. Highlight the first medication you wish to administer; then click the down arrow next to Select. From the drop-down menu, select **Administer** and complete the Administration Wizard by providing any information requested. When the Wizard stops asking for information, click **Administer to Patient**. Specify **Yes** when asked whether this administration should be recorded in the MAR. Finally, click **Finish**.

38 GETTING STARTED

■ **SELF-EVALUATION**

Now let's see how you did during your medication administration!

- Click on **Leave the Floor** at the bottom of your screen. From the Floor Menu, select **Look at Your Preceptor's Evaluation**. Then click on **Medication Scorecard**.

The following exercises will help you identify medication errors, investigate possible reasons for these errors, and reduce or prevent medication errors in the future.

1. Start by examining Table A. These are the medications you should have given to Dorothy Grant during this period of care. If each of the medications in Table A has a ✓ by it, then you made no errors. Congratulations!

If any medication has an X by it, then you made one or more medication errors.

Compare Tables A and B to determine which of the following types of errors you made: Wrong Dose, Wrong Route/Method/Site, or Wrong Time. Follow these steps:
   a. Find medications in Table A that were given incorrectly.
   b. Now see if those same medications are in Table B, which shows what you actually administered to Dorothy Grant.
   c. Comparing Tables A and B, match the Strength, Dose, Route/Method/Site, and Time for each medication you administered incorrectly.
   d. Then, using the form below, list the medications given incorrectly and mark the errors you made for each medication.

Medication	Strength	Dosage	Route	Method	Site	Time
	❏	❏	❏	❏	❏	❏
	❏	❏	❏	❏	❏	❏
	❏	❏	❏	❏	❏	❏
	❏	❏	❏	❏	❏	❏

2. To help you reduce future medication errors, consider the following list of possible reasons for errors.

   - Did not check drug against MAR for correct medication, correct dose, correct patient, correct route, correct time, correct documentation.
   - Did not check drug dose against MAR three times.
   - Did not open the unit dose package in the patient's room.
   - Did not correctly identify the patient using two identifiers.
   - Did not administer the drug on time.
   - Did not verify patient allergies.
   - Did not check the patient's current condition or vital sign parameters.
   - Did not consider why the patient would be receiving this drug.
   - Did not question why the drug was in the patient's drawer.
   - Did not check the physician's order and/or check with the pharmacist when there was a question about the drug or dose.
   - Did not verify that no adverse effects had occurred from a previous dose.

Copyright © 2011, 2007 by Mosby, Inc., an affiliate of Elsevier Inc. All rights reserved.

Based on the list of possibilities you just reviewed, determine how you made each error and record the reason in the form below:

Medication	Reason for Error

3. Look again at Table B. Are there medications listed that are not in Table A? If so, you gave a medication to Dorothy Grant that she should not have received. Complete the following exercises to help you understand how such an error might have been made.

   a. Perhaps you gave a medication that was on Dorothy Grant's MAR for this period of care, without recognizing that a change had occurred in the patient's condition, which should have caused you to reconsider. Review patient records as necessary and complete the following form:

Medication	Possible Reasons Not to Give This Medication

   b. Another possibility is that you gave Dorothy Grant a medication that should have been given at a different time. Check her MAR and complete the form below to determine whether you made a Wrong Time error:

Medication	Given to Dorothy Grant at What Time	Should Have Been Given at What Time

c. Maybe you gave another patient's medication to Dorothy Grant. In this case, you made a Wrong Patient error. Check the MARs of other patients and use the form below to determine whether you made this type of error:

Medication	Given to Dorothy Grant	Should Have Been Given to

4. The Medication Scorecard provides some other interesting sources of information. For example, if there is a medication selected for Dorothy Grant but it was not given to her, there will be an X by that medication in Table A, but it will not appear in Table B. In that case, you might have given this medication to some other patient, which is another type of Wrong Patient error. To investigate further, look at Table D, which lists the medications you gave to other patients. See whether you can find any medications ordered for Dorothy Grant that were given to another patient by mistake. However, before you make any decisions, be sure to cross-check the MAR for other patients because the same medication may have been ordered for multiple patients. Use the following form to record your findings:

Medication	Should Have Been Given to Dorothy Grant	Given by Mistake to

5. Now take some time to review the medication exercises you just completed. Use the form below to create an overall analysis of what you have learned. Once again, record each of the medication errors you made, including the type of each error. Then, for each error you made, indicate specifically what you would do differently to prevent this type of error from occurring again.

Medication	Type of Error	Error Prevention Tactic

Submit this form to your instructor if required as a graded assignment, or simply use these exercises to improve your understanding of medication errors and how to reduce them.

Name: _____   Date: _____

The following icons are used throughout this workbook to help you quickly identify particular activities and assignments:

 Indicates a reading assignment—tells you which textbook chapter(s) you should read before starting each lesson

 Indicates a writing activity

 Marks the beginning of an interactive virtual hospital activity—signals you to open or return to your *Virtual Clinical Excursions—Psychiatric* simulation

 Indicates additional virtual hospital activity instructions

 Indicates questions and activities that require you to consult your textbook

 Indicates the approximate time required to complete an exercise

LESSON 1

Psychotherapeutic Management in the Continuum of Care

Reading Assignment: Psychotherapeutic Management in the Continuum of Care (Chapter 2)

Patient: Harry George, Medical-Surgical Floor, Room 401

Goal: To understand the role of the nurse in caring for a patient along the continuum of care.

Objectives:

1. Describe the concept of the *continuum of care*.
2. Describe the components of the psychotherapeutic management model of nursing care.
3. Identify the elements of milieu management.
4. Compare and contrast the psychotherapeutic management model of caring for a patient in the hospital and in the community.

44 Virtual Clinical Excursions for Psychiatric Nursing

Exercise 1

 Writing Activity

 30 minutes

1. The continuum of care:
   a. provides a wide range of services based on the needs of the individual.
   b. provides levels of care in which the individual can move, depending on his or her needs.
   c. includes services from health promotion to prevention, treatment, rehabilitation, and recovery.
   d. provides care in a variety of treatment settings.
   e. includes all of the above.

2. The psychotherapeutic management model of nursing care includes which of the following components? Select all that apply.

   _____ Psychotherapy

   _____ Medication

   _____ Milieu management

   _____ Therapeutic nurse-patient relationship

   _____ Treating all patients alike

3. Milieu management, which consists of six elements, refers to a proactive approach that fosters a therapeutic environment in which patients can regain their health. Match each of the following milieu management elements with its description.

Element	Description
_____ Safety	a. Clear and enforceable behavioral limits
_____ Structure	b. Changing the environment to promote mental health
_____ Norms	c. Negotiating between dependence and independence
_____ Limit setting	d. The physical environment, schedule, and rules
_____ Balance	e. Behavioral expectations
_____ Environmental modification	f. Keeping the patient free from harm

Copyright © 2011, 2007 by Mosby, Inc., an affiliate of Elsevier Inc. All rights reserved.

4. Using the nurse-patient relationship intervention within the psychotherapeutic management model, describe the goals of a nurse working with a patient across the continuum of care from an acute care to a community setting.

Setting	Nurse-Patient Relationship Goals
Acute care hospital setting	
Community-based setting	

46 VIRTUAL CLINICAL EXCURSIONS FOR PSYCHIATRIC NURSING

Exercise 2

 Virtual Hospital Activity

 45 minutes

- Sign in to work at Pacific View Regional Hospital on the Medical-Surgical Floor for Period of Care 1. (*Note:* If you are already in the virtual hospital from a previous exercise, click on **Leave the Floor** and then on **Restart the Program** to get to the sign-in window.)
- From the Patient List, select Harry George (Room 401).
- Click on **Go to Nurses' Station**.
- Click on **Chart** and then on **401**.
- Click on the **History and Physical** and **Nursing Admission** tabs and review the information given.

1. Which of the following are stressors that have led to Harry George's current life situation? Select all that apply.

    _____ Motorcycle accident

    _____ Chronic bone infection in left foot

    _____ Estrangement from his wife and two sons

    _____ Loss of his job

    _____ Homelessness

    _____ Severe pain

2. Based on your review of the History and Physical and the Nursing Admission, list Harry George's medical diagnoses and the potential nursing problems associated with each.

Medical Diagnoses	**Nursing Problems**

3. Match each type of health education intervention with the corresponding specific health topic that Harry George will need to address during hospitalization and after discharge.

Type of Health Education Interventions

_____ Increase awareness of issues related to health and illness

_____ Increase understanding of potential stressors, possible outcomes, and alternative coping responses

_____ Increase knowledge of where and how to obtain resources

_____ Increase actual abilities

Specific Health Topic

a. Developing healthy coping skills such as stress reduction, motivation and self-esteem, problem solving, and stress management

b. Learning how becoming clean and sober, caring for self, managing pain and diabetes, and quitting smoking can positively affect health

c. Finding housing, finding/keeping job, and locating family members

d. Dealing with loss of family and job, homelessness, and pain

4. Considering Harry George's current living situation and 4-year history of alcoholism, if he were to try to quit drinking, what do you think would be the best type of program to accomplish this upon discharge?
   a. Community-based, sober-living house
   b. Inpatient alcohol/drug treatment program
   c. Outpatient visits with a drug/alcohol counselor
   d. Does not really matter because he will not stop drinking

5. What recovery challenges does Harry George face in each of the following areas of his life?

Area of Rehabilitation/Recovery	Challenges for Harry George
Activities of daily living (ADL)	
Interpersonal relationships	
Self-esteem	
Motivation	
Illness management	
Strengths	

LESSON 1—PSYCHOTHERAPEUTIC MANAGEMENT IN THE CONTINUUM OF CARE   49

6. What hospital-based resources are available to the nurse to help Harry George with community needs after discharge?

7. Using information from your text and taking into consideration Harry George's history and current needs, discuss how a positive change in his living/social environment could affect his rehabilitation and recovery.

LESSON **2**

The Nurse-Patient Relationship

Reading Assignment: Nurse-Patient Communication (Chapter 6)
Nurse-Patient Relationship (Chapter 7)

Patients: Jacquline Catanazaro, Medical-Surgical Floor, Room 402
Kathryn Doyle, Skilled Nursing Floor, Room 503

Goal: To demonstrate the importance of the therapeutic nurse-patient relationship and to identify and use therapeutic communication techniques with patients.

Objectives:

1. Distinguish therapeutic communication from social communication.
2. Identify the characteristics of therapeutic listening.
3. Discuss the importance of empathy in the therapeutic nurse-patient relationship.
4. Identify the stages of a therapeutic nurse-patient relationship.
5. Understand common nurse-patient relationship challenges that may impede a patient's progress toward treatment goals.
6. Observe and identify effective communication techniques used by the nurse in nurse-patient interactions.

Exercise 1

 Writing Activity

 30 minutes

1. The following characteristics apply to either therapeutic or social communication. Match each characteristic with the type of communications to which it corresponds.

   Characteristic

   _____ Focuses on helping another

   _____ Involves equal disclosure of personal information and intimacy

   _____ Planned and directed by the nurse

   _____ Relies on patient's disclosures

   _____ Allows both parties equal opportunities for spontaneity

   _____ Includes mutual confidentiality

   _____ Involves sharing information with the treatment team

   _____ Involves both participants seeking to have needs met

   Type of Communication

   a. Therapeutic communication

   b. Social communication

2. Therapeutic listening, an important component of the therapeutic use of self, is composed of which of the following attributes? Select all that apply.

   _____ Using eye contact

   _____ Being relaxed

   _____ Being patient

   _____ Asking questions

   _____ Offering empathy and support

   _____ Summarizing important points

   _____ Looking away often to appear detached

   _____ Responding verbally and nonverbally to encourage patient to continue

   _____ Sitting in a closed position

3. Empathy is an essential skill of the psychiatric nurse. Which of the following describes empathy?
   a. Recognizes and understands the patient's feelings and points of view objectively
   b. Conveys caring, compassion, and concern for the patient
   c. Helps patient be more accepting of his or her feelings
   d. Assists the patient to express feelings more readily
   e. All of the above

4. The therapeutic nurse-patient relationship has three stages. List the most important characteristics of each stage in the table below.

Stage	Characteristics
Stage I: Orientation	
Stage II: Working	
Stage III: Termination	

5. The nurse may encounter symptoms of mental illness that present challenges in working with a patient. List several symptoms that you would consider challenges in terms of the nurse-patient relationship.

LESSON 2—THE NURSE-PATIENT RELATIONSHIP 55

Exercise 2

 Virtual Hospital Activity

 45 minutes

- Sign in to work at Pacific View Regional Hospital on the Medical-Surgical Floor for Period of Care 1. (*Note:* If you are already in the virtual hospital from a previous exercise, click on **Leave the Floor** and then on **Restart the Program** to get to the sign-in window.)
- From the Patient List, select Jacquline Catanazaro (Room 402).
- Click on **Go to Nurses' Station** and then on **402** at the bottom of the screen.
- Click on **Patient Care** and then on **Nurse-Client Interactions**.
- Select and view the video titled **0730: Intervention—Airway**. (*Note:* Check the virtual clock to see whether enough time has elapsed. You can use the fast-forward feature to advance the time by 2-minute intervals if the video is not yet available. Then click again on **Patient Care** and **Nurse-Client Interactions** to refresh the screen.)

 1. As you watch the 0730 video, make note of the types of therapeutic verbal and nonverbal communication techniques the nurse uses. Record these in the first column of the table below. Then, in the second column, list specific examples of verbal and nonverbal communication used by the nurse that demonstrate each technique. (*Hint:* See pages 64-65 in your textbook.)

	Therapeutic Communication Techniques Used by Nurse	Specific Examples of Nurse Communication
Verbal		
Nonverbal		

56 VIRTUAL CLINICAL EXCURSIONS FOR PSYCHIATRIC NURSING

Now let's jump ahead in time to observe a later interaction between the nurse and this patient.

- Click on **Leave the Floor** and then on **Restart the Program**.
- Sign in to work at Pacific View Regional Hospital on the Medical-Surgical Floor for Period of Care 2.
- From the Patient List, select Jacquline Catanazaro (Room 402).
- Click on **Go to Nurses' Station** and then on **402** at the bottom of the screen.
- Click on **Patient Care** and then on **Nurse-Client Interactions**.
- Select and view the video titled **1115: Assessment—Readiness to Learn**. (*Note:* Check the virtual clock to see whether enough time has elapsed. You can use the fast-forward feature to advance the time by 2-minute intervals if the video is not yet available. Then click again on **Patient Care** and **Nurse-Client Interactions** to refresh the screen.)

2. As you observe the 1115 video, make note of the types of therapeutic verbal and nonverbal communication techniques the nurse uses. Record these in the first column below. Then, in the second column, list specific examples of verbal and nonverbal communication used by the nurse that demonstrate each technique. (*Hint:* See pages 64-65 in your textbook.)

Therapeutic Communication Techniques Used by Nurse	Specific Examples of Nurse Communication

Verbal

Nonverbal

Next, let's look at an interaction between the nurse and a different patient.

- Click on **Leave the Floor** and then on **Restart the Program**.
- Sign in to work at Pacific View Regional Hospital on the Skilled Nursing Floor for Period of Care 1.
- From the Patient List, select Kathryn Doyle (Room 503).
- Click on **Go to Nurses' Station** and then on **503** at the bottom of the screen.
- Click on **Patient Care** and then on **Nurse-Client Interactions**.
- Select and view the video titled **0730: Assessment—Biopsychosocial**. (*Note:* Check the virtual clock to see whether enough time has elapsed. You can use the fast-forward feature to advance the time by 2-minute intervals if the video is not yet available. Then click again on **Patient Care** and **Nurse-Client Interactions** to refresh the screen.)

3. As you observe the 0730 video, make note of types of therapeutic verbal and nonverbal communication techniques the nurse uses. Record these in the first column below. Then, in the second column, list specific examples of verbal and nonverbal communication used by the nurse that demonstrate each technique. (*Hint:* See pages 64-65 in your textbook.)

Therapeutic Communication Techniques Used by Nurse	Specific Examples of Nurse Communication

Verbal

Nonverbal

LESSON 3

Nursing Process

Reading Assignment: Nursing Process (Chapter 8)

Patient: Harry George, Medical-Surgical Floor, Room 401

Goal: To understand the role of the nurse in caring for a complex patient using the nursing process.

Objectives:

1. Identify the phases in the nursing process.
2. Discuss the components included in the nursing assessment.
3. Use assessment data to formulate a plan of care.
4. Describe three types of formats for treatment planning.
5. Write clear, specific, measurable outcome statements in a plan of care.
6. Use the nursing process in caring for a complex patient.
7. Discuss the nurse's involvement in discharge.

Exercise 1

 Writing Activity

 45 minutes

1. In caring for patients, the professional nurse uses a six-step nursing process. Match the following columns to show the correct order of the phases of the nursing process.

Nursing Process Phase	Name
_____ Phase I	a. Intervention
_____ Phase II	b. Outcome identification
_____ Phase III	c. Assessment
_____ Phase IV	d. Evaluation
_____ Phase V	e. Planning
_____ Phase VI	f. Nursing diagnosis

2. An important component of the initial assessment is the mental status examination, which focuses on the patient's current state in terms of _____, _____, and _____.

3. The psychiatric assessment includes both mental status and psychosocial components. It is important for the nurse to understand elements within each of these components. Match each specific aspect of the psychiatric assessment below to its corresponding component.

Specific Aspect	Component of Psychiatric Assessment
_____ General appearance	a. Mental status
_____ Behavior and motor activity	b. Psychosocial
_____ Admission data and reason for admission	
_____ Support systems	
_____ Mood, affect, and speech patterns	
_____ Previous mental health history and treatment	
_____ Cultural and spiritual aspects	
_____ Thought clarity, content, and processes	
_____ Insight, judgment, and motivation	
_____ Orientation to time, place, and person	
_____ Current medical problems and medications	

4. From data gathered in the assessment, the nurse makes a nursing diagnosis. Which of the following are correct statements regarding nursing diagnoses? Select all that apply.

   _____ Nursing diagnoses are statements that describe an individual's potential or actual problems.

   _____ Nursing diagnoses are not as relevant as medical diagnoses.

   _____ Nursing diagnoses include contributing or causative factors.

   _____ Nursing diagnoses should be specific and indicate behavioral outcomes.

5. Outcome statements, or goals, are measurable and achievable and consist of adaptive behaviors to replace dysfunctional ones. Explain why outcome statements are such an important part of the nursing process.

6. In the planning phase of the nursing process, the nurse often uses standardized nursing care plans, also called _____,

   _____, or

   _____.

7. During the planning phase of the nursing process, nursing interventions are developed. Which of the following statements regarding nursing interventions are correct? Select all that apply.

   _____ Nursing interventions focus on safety, structure, support, and symptom management.

   _____ Nursing interventions are used to guide patients in solving problems for themselves.

   _____ Nursing interventions are always written in clear, specific, and measurable language.

   _____ Nursing interventions are selected to achieve patient outcomes.

   _____ Nursing interventions are individualized to specific patient's needs.

8. Describe the two types of evaluation the nurse uses during the evaluation phase of the nursing process.

64 VIRTUAL CLINICAL EXCURSIONS FOR PSYCHIATRIC NURSING

Exercise 2

 Virtual Hospital Activity

 30 minutes

- Sign in to work at Pacific View Regional Hospital on the Medical-Surgical Floor for Period of Care 3. (*Note:* If you are already in the virtual hospital from a previous exercise, click on **Leave the Floor** and then on **Restart the Program** to get to the sign-in window.)
- From the Patient List, select Harry George (Room 401).
- Click on **Go to Nurses' Station**.
- Click on **Chart** and then on **401**.
- Click on the **History and Physical** and **Nursing Admission** tabs and review the information given.

1. Based on the History and Physical and the Nursing Admission, what data do you believe are most important for the nurse in making a nursing diagnosis?

- Click on the **Mental Health** tab and review the Psychiatric/Mental Health Assessment.
- Click on the **Consultations** tab and review the Psychiatric Consult.

2. List any additional mental status and psychosocial data that these documents provide.

3. List some examples of potential nursing diagnoses that may correspond to Harry George's medical diagnoses below.

Medical Diagnoses	Nursing Diagnoses
Major depressive disorder	
Substance abuse	

4. The initial treatment plan begins with identifying one or two of the patient's most critical problems that need to be addressed immediately. In considering Harry George's mental health issues, what are his most critical needs?
    a. Feeling anxious and overwhelmed
    b. Alcohol abuse and hopelessness
    c. Social isolation and loneliness
    d. Homelessness

5. Write a clear, specific, and measurable outcome statement related to the nursing problems of restlessness, agitation, and combativeness.

6. According to the psychiatric consultation in Harry George's chart, which of the following are included in the treatment plan to help Harry George meet his goals while he is hospitalized and after he is discharged? Select all that apply.

   _____ Initiate sertraline, an antianxiety/antidepressant medication.

   _____ Initiate a comprehensive alcohol/drug treatment program.

   _____ Begin cognitive therapy for depression.

   _____ It does not really matter since he will not be able to stop drinking.

   _____ Begin vocational rehabilitation skill training.

   _____ Offer support to find housing.

7. Nurses are expected to participate in writing a discharge summary and to provide the patient with discharge instructions. Below are elements that would be included in Harry George's discharge summary/instructions. Match each element with the discharge document in which it would be recorded.

   Critical Element

   _____ Vital signs and blood glucose level

   _____ Behavior and attitude on discharge

   _____ Dressing and wound care instructions

   _____ Referrals to other services in hospital and community

   _____ Follow-up appointments: type, names, dates, and times

   _____ Progress on problems while in hospital

   _____ Patient's signature verifying that he is able read and understands the instructions

   _____ Medications: names, dosages, and times

   _____ Educational materials

   _____ Risk assessment, danger to self

   Discharge Document

   a. Discharge summary

   b. Discharge instructions

LESSON 4

Stress, Anxiety, Coping, and Crisis

Reading Assignment: Stress, Anxiety, Coping, and Crisis (Chapter 9)

Patient: Dorothy Grant, Obstetrics Floor, Room 201

Goal: To care for a patient on an obstetrics floor who is experiencing stress and anxiety as a result of a crisis.

Objectives:

1. Explain the relationship among stress, anxiety, coping, and crisis.
2. Describe two types of stressors.
3. Identify the characteristics of anxiety.
4. List the NANDA diagnoses for anxiety, coping, and crisis.
5. Match specific nursing interventions with each level of anxiety presented.
6. Show the sequence of crisis intervention strategies.
7. Identify needs for a patient in crisis who is experiencing anxiety.
8. Develop treatment interventions and outcomes for a patient with anxiety.

Exercise 1

 Writing Activity

 30 minutes

1. Explain the relationship among stress, anxiety, coping, and crisis.

2. Define maturational and situational stressors and give an example of each type.

3. Anxiety can be described in a variety of ways. Which of the following are valid descriptions or characteristics of anxiety? Select all that apply.

   _____ Emotional response that triggers behavior

   _____ Apprehension

   _____ Fearfulness

   _____ Sense of powerlessness resulting from a threat

   _____ Objective experience

   _____ Physical pain

4. Which of the following are NANDA diagnoses related to anxiety, coping, and crisis? Select all that apply.

   _____ Anxiety

   _____ Depression

   _____ Posttraumatic stress syndrome

   _____ Ineffective coping

   _____ Social isolation

5. In working with a patient experiencing anxiety, the nurse must correlate interventions with the patient's level of anxiety. Match each nursing intervention listed below with the level of anxiety to which it would apply.

	Nursing Intervention	**Level of Anxiety**
_____	Decrease anxiety; use kind, firm, simple directions; use time-outs; provide IM medication	a. Mild
_____	Guide firmly or physically take control; give IM medication; use seclusion and/or restraints	b. Moderate
_____	Discuss sources of anxiety; assist with problem solving	c. Severe
_____	Encourage venting, crying, exercise, relaxation; offer PO medication	d. Panic

6. Methods of coping can be placed into four categories according to their levels of effectiveness in decreasing anxiety or eliminating the source of anxiety. Match each method of coping below to its correct description.

   Method of Coping

   _____ Adaptive

   _____ Palliative

   _____ Maladaptive

   _____ Dysfunctional

   Description

   a. Not successful in reducing anxiety or solving the problem. Minimal functioning is difficult and new problems develop.

   b. Temporarily decreases anxiety but does not solve the problem, so the anxiety gradually returns. The brief relief allows the patient to problem-solve.

   c. Solves the problem that is causing the anxiety, so the anxiety is decreased.

   d. Attempts (unsuccessfully) to decrease anxiety without attempting to solve the problem; therefore the anxiety continues.

7. Place the following crisis intervention strategies in the correct order of priority.

   Order of Priority

   _____ First

   _____ Second

   _____ Third

   _____ Fourth

   _____ Fifth

   Crisis Intervention Strategy

   a. Make arrangements for follow-up care

   b. Focus on strengths and adaptive coping

   c. Reestablish equilibrium and stabilization

   d. Prevent harm to self, harm to others, and further decompensation

   e. Offer suggestions for concrete instructions and specific problem solving

LESSON 4—STRESS, ANXIETY, COPING, AND CRISIS   71

Exercise 2

 Virtual Hospital Activity

 45 minutes

- Sign in to work at Pacific View Regional Hospital on the Obstetrics Floor for Period of Care 1. (*Note:* If you are already in the virtual hospital from a previous exercise, click on **Leave the Floor** and then on **Restart the Program** to get to the sign-in window.)
- From the Patient List, select Dorothy Grant (Room 401).
- Click on **Get Report** and read the Clinical Report.

    1. According to the change-of-shift report, what level of anxiety is Dorothy Grant experiencing?
        a. Mild
        b. Moderate
        c. Severe
        d. Panic

    2. Dorothy Grant's concerns about safety for _____ and

        _____ are causing her anxiety.

 - Click on **Go to Nurses' Station**; then click on **201** at the bottom of the screen.
- Read the **Initial Observations**.

    3. How does the nurse's assessment of Dorothy Grant's anxiety level in the Initial Observations compare with the assessment in the change-of-shift report?

 - Click on **Chart** and then on **201**.
- Click on the **Nursing Admission** tab and review the information given.

    4. What are two stressors listed that contribute to Dorothy Grant's anxiety?

5. Dorothy Grant has experienced traumatic injury by her husband. What are your reactions (thoughts and feelings) regarding this event?

6. Which of the following outcome statements best fit Dorothy Grant's treatment plan? Select all that apply.

_____ Demonstrates enhanced ability to problem-solve and make decisions

_____ Demonstrates ability to function in a mild anxiety state

_____ Demonstrates effective coping skills

_____ Demonstrates concern for personal safety by starting to verbalize worries

7. You have assessed that Dorothy Grant's level of anxiety is moderate. Using strategies presented in Chapter 9 of your textbook, develop nursing interventions based on each of the following aspects of treatment.

Aspect of Treatment	Nursing Interventions
Recognition of problem	
Insight into her situation and resulting anxiety	
Education about her situation	
Coping with her situation	

LESSON 5

Cultural Competence and Spirituality

Reading Assignment: Cultural Competence in Psychiatric Nursing (Chapter 14)
Spirituality (Chapter 15)

Patient: Carlos Reyes, Skilled Nursing Floor, Room 504

Goal: To understand cultural and spiritual aspects of psychiatric nursing care.

Objectives:

1. Understand how culture helps define mental health.
2. Discuss how the DSM IV-TR addresses culture and spiritual beliefs.
3. Define culturally competent care.
4. Examine practice barriers and methods to work through them in order to provide culturally competent care.
5. Describe culturally competent nursing care.
6. Identify the four primary worldviews and their relevance in the provision of culturally competent care.
7. Identify the basic elements in a cultural assessment.
8. List the four spiritual themes that patients with psychiatric illness seek.
9. Provide the rationale for having a professional chaplain on the psychiatric treatment team.
10. Provide care for a patient in the Hispanic culture.

Exercise 1

 Writing Activity

 30 minutes

1. Discuss how the DSM IV-TR addresses syndromes unique to specific cultures and how culture and religious/spiritual beliefs might influence the level of compliance with treatment.

2. Which of the following statements accurately describes how culture influences an individual's mental health? Select all that apply.

    _____ Each cultural group has beliefs, values, and practices that guide its members in ways of thinking and acting.

    _____ The framework that describes mental health and illness is based on Eastern thought.

    _____ Cultural differences deem what behavior is normal and what behavior is aberrant.

    _____ The influence of a culture is so pervasive that people can fail to recognize cultural aspects of life.

    _____ Culture is irrelevant when it comes to treating symptoms of mental illness.

3. In providing care to culturally diverse populations, the nurse will encounter difficulties in practice and must be knowledgeable about methods to overcome these difficulties. Listed below are three cultural practice issues and their associated difficulties. Complete the table by giving examples of how the nurse can work through each issue and overcome the barriers.

Cultural Practice Issue	Barriers	Examples for Overcoming Barriers
Communication	Miscommunication due to differences in spoken language and in the meaning of nonverbal communication	
Assessment	Failure to assess the patient's cultural perspective using available clinical cultural assessment tools	
Values and beliefs	Lack of knowledge and sensitivity regarding the patient's beliefs and practices; patient may be unaware of the nurse's cultural perspective	
Ethnopharmacology	Genetic variations in drug metabolism found in people of all ethnicities	

4. In reference to the culturally competent psychiatric nurse, indicate whether each statement below is true or false.

   a. _____ Shows proficiency in cultural awareness, knowledge, and skills to promote effective health care

   b. _____ Has knowledge about the process of cultural competence

   c. _____ Incorporates concept into interactions with peers, students, patients, families, and communities

   d. _____ Uses cultural competence to enhance clinical excellence and promote recovery of the psychiatric patient

5. It is important that the nurse understand an individual patient's worldview because it influences health care beliefs and actions. Match each of the four primary worldviews below to its corresponding characteristics.

Worldview	Characteristics
_____ Analytic	a. Belief in spirituality and significance of relationships and interactions; learning style is through verbal communication.
_____ Relational	
_____ Community	b. Belief that a form of interconnectedness exists between human beings and the earth and that individuals need to take care of the earth.
_____ Ecologic	

  c. Values detail to time, individuality, and possessions; style of learning is through written, hands-on, and visual resources.

  d. Believes that community needs and concerns are more important than individual ones; learning style involves quiet, respectful communication, meditation, and reading.

6. List the basic elements that nurses must include in their cultural assessment of a patient.

7. When asked, most psychiatric patients state they want to be asked whether they have a religious preference and want the nurse to contact a member from the cultural group with which they identify. This is true because many patients want to talk to someone who can provide the four essential spiritual themes:

   _____, _____,

   _____, and _____.

8. Discuss the importance of having a professional chaplain on the psychiatric treatment team.

80 VIRTUAL CLINICAL EXCURSIONS FOR PSYCHIATRIC NURSING

Exercise 2

 Virtual Hospital Activity

 45 minutes

- Sign in to work at Pacific View Regional Hospital on the Skilled Nursing Floor for Period of Care 1. (*Note:* If you are already in the virtual hospital from a previous exercise, click on **Leave the Floor** and then on **Restart the Program** to get to the sign-in window.)
- From the Patient List, select Carlos Reyes (Room 504).
- Click on **Go to Nurses' Station**.
- Click on **Chart** and then on **504**.
- Click on the **History and Physical** and **Nursing Admission** tabs and review the information given.

1. According to the information in his chart, Carlos Reyes' ethnicity is identified as

   _____ and his religion is listed as _____.

2. In order to perform a cultural assessment on Carlos Reyes, there are several key questions that are important to include. Which of the following should be included? Select all that apply. (*Hint:* Review Chapter 14 in your textbook.)

   _____ Where were you born?

   _____ What is your primary language?

   _____ Would you like an interpreter?

   _____ Is there anyone you want me to contact?

   _____ How is your illness viewed by your culture?

   _____ What is your age?

   _____ How tall are you?

   _____ What do you weigh?

   _____ Do you have a religious preference?

   _____ What do you do to get better when you are medically ill? Mentally ill?

   _____ Are there any special foods you like to eat?

   _____ Are there certain medications or herbs you are taking?

Copyright © 2011, 2007 by Mosby, Inc., an affiliate of Elsevier Inc. All rights reserved.

3. What are some characteristics of the Hispanic culture?

4. Discuss the cultural factors relevant in caring for Carlos Reyes.

82 Virtual Clinical Excursions for Psychiatric Nursing

- Click on **Return to Nurses' Station** and then on **504** at the bottom of the screen.
- Click on **Patient Care** and then on **Nurse-Client Interactions**.
- Select and view the video titled **0740: Drowsiness—Contributing Factor**. (*Note:* Check the virtual clock to see whether enough time has elapsed. You can use the fast-forward feature to advance the time by 2-minute intervals if the video is not yet available. Then click again on **Patient Care** and **Nurse-Client Interactions** to refresh the screen.)

5. What two interventions did the nurse implement to address Carlos Reyes' son's concerns about his father's drowsiness?

6. What other actions could the nurse have taken?

- Click on **Patient Care** and then on **Nurse-Client Interactions**.
- Select and view the video titled **0745: Family Teaching—Medication**. (*Note:* Check the virtual clock to see whether enough time has elapsed. You can use the fast-forward feature to advance the time by 2-minute intervals if the video is not yet available. Then click again on **Patient Care** and **Nurse-Client Interactions** to refresh the screen.)
- Click on the **Drug** icon in the lower left corner and search for oxazepam.

7. What is the indication of oxazepam?

LESSON 5—CULTURAL COMPETENCE AND SPIRITUALITY   83

8. What is oxazepam's effect on brain function?

9. Identify the side effect of oxazepam that is concerning Carlos Reyes' son.

→ • Click on **Patient Care** and then on **Nurse-Client Interactions**.
  • Select and view the video titled **0750: Assessment—Level of Assistance**. (*Note:* Check the virtual clock to see whether enough time has elapsed. You can use the fast-forward feature to advance the time by 2-minute intervals if the video is not yet available. Then click again on **Patient Care** and **Nurse-Client Interactions** to refresh the screen.)

  10. Which of the following aspects of the mental status exam is the nurse attempting to assess? Select all that apply.

      _____ Appearance

      _____ Speech

      _____ Motor activity

      _____ Interaction

      _____ Level of consciousness

      _____ Emotional state: mood and affect

Copyright © 2011, 2007 by Mosby, Inc., an affiliate of Elsevier Inc. All rights reserved.

11. Assess the level of assistance that Carlos Reyes will need in order to sit up and eat his breakfast. What is the role of Carlos Reyes' family at mealtime?

LESSON 6

Schizophrenia

Reading Assignment: Schizophrenia and Other Psychoses (Chapter 27)

Patient: Jacquline Catanazaro, Medical-Surgical Floor, Room 402

Goal: To care for a patient with chronic schizophrenia who is hospitalized for acute asthma.

Objectives:

1. Define *schizophrenia*.
2. Discuss the prevalence and characteristics of schizophrenia in the population.
3. List the positive and negative symptoms of schizophrenia.
4. Understand the difference between objective signs and subjective symptoms of schizophrenia.
5. List potential stressors that can produce a relapse of patients with schizophrenia.
6. Identify communication techniques for patients exhibiting hallucinations and delusions.
7. Describe the importance of education as part of the treatment for patients with schizophrenia and their family.
8. Discuss aspects of treatment across the continuum of care for a patient with schizophrenia.
9. Explain the importance of relapse prevention for a patient with schizophrenia.
10. Discuss medication as a treatment for patients diagnosed with schizophrenia.

Exercise 1

 Writing Activity

 45 minutes

1. Schizophrenia is a brain disease classified as a major psychotic disorder characterized by

    disturbances in _____, thought processes,

    _____, feeling, _____, attention, and

    _____.

2. The impact of schizophrenia on individuals and society is enormous. Which of the following statements are true about the prevalence and characteristics of schizophrenia in the population? Select all that apply.

    _____ Men and women are equally represented in the population of individuals with schizophrenia.

    _____ Of people diagnosed with schizophrenia, 100% have the disease for life.

    _____ The most typical onset for schizophrenia is between the ages of 15-25.

    _____ Men have a more severe course; women have more positive symptoms.

    _____ Substance abuse disorders occur in approximately 40%-50% of individuals with schizophrenia.

    _____ Only upper middle-class individuals suffer from schizophrenia.

    _____ Approximately 1% of Americans will experience schizophrenia in their lifetime.

3. It is important to understand the positive and negative symptoms of schizophrenia. List the positive and negative symptoms associated with each category below.

Category	Positive Symptoms	Negative Symptoms
Thinking		
Emotion		
Speech		
Behavior		

4. Communicating with a patient who has schizophrenia can be challenging. In the table below, list at least three communication techniques that are effective to use with patients experiencing the positive symptoms of hallucinations and delusions.

Positive Symptom	Communication Techniques
Hallucinations	
Delusions	

5. In addition to the positive and negative symptoms discussed above, there are also objective signs (apparent to others) and subjective symptoms (internally felt) of schizophrenia. Identify each sign/symptom below as either objective or subjective.

Signs/Symptoms	Sign/Symptom Category
____ Alterations in personal relationships	a. Objective
____ Altered perception	b. Subjective
____ Altered consciousness	
____ Alterations of thought	
____ Alterations of activity	
____ Alterations in affect	

6. According to the vulnerability-stress model, stressful events can precipitate a new episode or exacerbation of the symptoms of schizophrenia. Select all stressors that you think could lead to a relapse in an individual with schizophrenia.

   _____ Low self-concept/self-confidence

   _____ Lack of social support; estranged from family

   _____ Housing difficulties; living in impoverished area

   _____ Aggressive/violent behavior; crime in neighborhood

   _____ Lack of sleep; poor nutrition

   _____ Poor medication management; stops taking medication

   _____ Lack of transportation

   _____ Not enough money to buy needed items

   _____ Job pressures; trouble finding work

   _____ Interpersonal difficulties; inability to express self

   _____ Social isolation; loneliness

7. Discuss the importance of involving the patient and the patient's family in the treatment process.

8. Patients with schizophrenia are treated across the continuum of care. This continuum of care includes which of the following? Select all that apply.

   _____ Hospitalization for acute symptoms

   _____ Long-term hospitalization for those who are resistant to treatment

   _____ Day treatment or similar community programs for patients needing to stabilize symptoms

   _____ Supportive housing for those who cannot live with their families

Exercise 2

 Virtual Hospital Activity

 45 minutes

- Sign in to work at Pacific View Regional Hospital on the Medical-Surgical Floor for Period of Care 3. (*Note:* If you are already in the virtual hospital from a previous exercise, click on **Leave the Floor** and then on **Restart the Program** to get to the sign-in window.)
- From the Patient List, select Jacquline Catanazaro (Room 402).
- Click on **Go to Nurses' Station**.
- Click on **Chart** and then on **402**.
- Click on the **Nurse's Notes** tab and read the notes for Monday at 1600.

1. Which of the following pieces of information in the Nurse's Notes have implications for discharge planning? Select all that apply.

   _____ Patient has asthma.

   _____ Sister is patient's main support.

   _____ Patient has no transportation.

   _____ Patient has a history of stopping her psychiatric medication.

- Read the **Nurse's Notes** for Tuesday at 0400.

2. Jacquline Catanazaro's statement that people are putting poison into her IV is an example of which of the following types of delusion?
   a. Grandiose
   b. Persecutory
   c. Paranoid
   d. None of the above

- Read the **Nurse's Notes** for Wednesday at 0600.

3. This note describes symptoms of schizophrenia that have a direct relationship to Jacquline Catanazaro's asthma. Explain this relationship.

92   VIRTUAL CLINICAL EXCURSIONS FOR PSYCHIATRIC NURSING

→ • Click on the **Consultations** tab and review the Psychiatric Consult.

4. The positive symptom of schizophrenia that is described in the report is

   _____. The negative symptoms described are social

   _____ and low _____.

5. The plan outlined in the Psychiatric Consult includes exercise and nutrition. Comment on the relevance of diet and exercise as part of the plan of care for Jacquline Catanazaro.

→ • Click on the **History and Physical** and **Nursing Admission** tabs and review the information given.

6. Relapse can be a devastating part of the disease of schizophrenia. For each category below and on the next page, list Jacquline Catanazaro's barriers to compliance that may result in future relapses.

Category	Barriers to Compliance
Health	

Thoughts

Category	Barriers to Compliance
Attitudes	
Behavior	
Socialization	
Medication	

7. Education will be a critical component of Jacquline Catanazaro's treatment plan. Which of the following are educational needs for Jacquline Catanazaro? Select all that apply.

   _____ Education on healthy living

   _____ Medication knowledge and management

   _____ Psychoeducation on her illness

   _____ Symptom management

   _____ Preventing relapse

- Click on **Return to Nurses' Station**.
- Click on **MAR** and then on **402**.
- Scroll down to locate the antipsychotic medication ordered for Jacquline Catanazaro.
- Click on **Return to Nurses' Station**.
- Click on the **Drug** icon in the lower left corner of the screen and review the antipsychotic medication that you identified in the MAR.

8. Complete the table below based on your review of the information in the Drug Guide.

Name of medication

Indication

Mechanism of action

Side effects

Dosage

Nursing considerations

Patient teaching

LESSON 6—SCHIZOPHRENIA   95

9. Compare the medication dosage that Jacquline Catanazaro is receiving with the usual dosage outlined in the Drug Guide. What might be the rationale for the current dosage that the physician has prescribed for Jacquline Catanazaro?

- Click on **Return to Nurses' Station** and then on **402** at the bottom of the screen.
- Click on **Patient Care** and then on **Nurse-Client Interactions**.
- Select and view the video titled **1500: Intervention—Patient Teaching**. (*Note:* Check the virtual clock to see whether enough time has elapsed. You can use the fast-forward feature to advance the time by 2-minute intervals if the video is not yet available. Then click again on **Patient Care** and **Nurse-Client Interactions** to refresh the screen.)
- Now select and view the video titled **1540: Discharge Planning**. (*Note:* Check the virtual clock to see whether enough time has elapsed. You can use the fast-forward feature to advance the time by 2-minute intervals if the video is not yet available. Then click again on **Patient Care** and **Nurse-Client Interactions** to refresh the screen.)

10. Discuss the importance of including Jacquline Catanazaro's sister in the discharge planning and relapse prevention process.

LESSON 7

Depression

Reading Assignment: Depression (Chapter 28)

Patient: Kelly Brady, Obstetrics Floor, Room 203

Goal: To care for a patient experiencing a medical health crisis who also has symptoms of depression.

Objectives:

1. Understand the prevalence and occurrence of depression.
2. Describe common risk factors and precipitating stressors in depression.
3. Identify symptoms associated with depression.
4. Determine the elements to include in a suicide risk assessment for a patient with depression.
5. Plan for relapse prevention for a patient with depression.
6. Develop a treatment plan for a patient with depression.
7. Examine the relationship between depression and pregnancy.
8. Describe effective treatments including pharmacologic treatment for depressed patients.
9. Identify realistic discharge criteria for a patient with depression.

98 Virtual Clinical Excursions for Psychiatric Nursing

Exercise 1

 Writing Activity

 45 minutes

1. Mood disorders, particularly depression, are common. Which of the following statements are correct regarding depression? Select all that apply.

    _____ Major depressive disorders are about twice as common in women as in men.

    _____ Depression occurs more frequently in Caucasian and Hispanic females and in African-American males.

    _____ Almost 17% of Americans will develop a major depression in their lifetime.

    _____ 30 million people are affected by depression at any given time in the United States.

    _____ The average age for the adult onset of depression is the mid- to late 20s.

    _____ Having a positive family history for depression increases one's risk for depression.

2. Depression may result from a complex interaction of causes and common risk factors. Which of the following causes/risk factors can contribute to depression? Select all that apply.

    _____ Early debilitating life experiences, such as parental losses or inconsistent parenting

    _____ Family history of depressive disorders, especially first-degree relatives; history of family member suicide

    _____ Brain chemistry abnormalities

    _____ Active alcohol/substance abuse

    _____ Postpartum

    _____ Medical illnesses such as CNS, metabolic, endocrine, and neoplastic disorders, collagen vascular diseases, and certain infections

    _____ Lack of social support

3. Complete the table below by listing examples of symptoms associated with major depression.

Type of Symptom	Examples
Affective/emotional	
Behavioral	
Cognitive	
Social	

4. While assessing a patient with depression, it is important to think about safety first. Explain the actions that the nurse should take to ensure the patient's safety.

5. People with depression have a genuine need to believe that things can get better. Which of the following interventions can help patients with this belief? Select all that apply.

   _____ The nurse should initially express hope to the patient.

   _____ The nurse should reinforce the fact that depression is a self-limiting disorder and the future will be better.

   _____ The nurse should explain to the patient that depression is a chronic disease.

6. What are some important interventions that the nurse should employ when working with a depressed patient?

7. Considering what we know about the clinical course of depression, which of the following measure(s) do you think will help in preventing recurrence?
   a. Education regarding symptom recognition and seeking help early
   b. Lifetime monitoring and maintenance
   c. Adhering to the treatment regime
   d. Medication, psychotherapy, and self-help strategies
   e. All of the above

8. Successful behavior is a powerful tool to counteract depression. List specific interventions the nurse can use with a depressed patient to effect positive behavioral change, including possible activities that the patient can accomplish in order to make positive behavioral changes.

9. For treating patients with depression, which of the following classes of medications has proven to be the most effective with the fewest side effects?
   a. Selective serotonin reuptake inhibitors (SSRIs)
   b. Monoamine oxidase inhibitors (MAOIs)
   c. Tricyclic antidepressant drugs (TCAs)

10. Discuss reasons that the nurse should educate a depressed patient on the illness of depression and self-management strategies.

102 Virtual Clinical Excursions for Psychiatric Nursing

Exercise 2

 Virtual Hospital Activity

 30 minutes

- Sign in to work at Pacific View Regional Hospital on the Obstetrics Floor for Period of Care 1. (*Note:* If you are already in the virtual hospital from a previous exercise, click on **Leave the Floor** and then on **Restart the Program** to get to the sign-in window.)
- From the Patient List, select Kelly Brady (Room 203).
- Click on **Go to Nurses' Station** and then on **203** at the bottom of the screen.
- Read the **Initial Observations**.
- Click on **Patient Care**.
- Click on **Head & Neck** and then on **Mental Status** and review the assessment data.

1. During Kelly Brady's mental status assessment, the two documented behavioral symptoms

   of depression are _____ and high _____.

- Click on **Chart** and then on **203**.
- Click on the **History and Physical** tab and review the information given.

2. Kelly Brady's depression follows the typical clinical course for depression. Which of the following statements apply to Kelly Brady's recurrence of depression? Select all that apply.

   _____ Two-thirds of people with depression have a second occurrence within 10 years.

   _____ Recurrent episodes of depression tend to be increasingly intense.

   _____ There tend to be shorter time periods between recurrent episodes of depression.

3. What is the predisposing factor in Kelly Brady's family history related to depression?

4. What is the key factor in Kelly Brady's own past medical history related to depression?

Copyright © 2011, 2007 by Mosby, Inc., an affiliate of Elsevier Inc. All rights reserved.

LESSON 7—DEPRESSION 103

- Click on **Return to Room 203**.
- Click on **Leave the Floor** and then on **Restart the Program**.
- Sign in to work on the Obstetrics Floor for Period of Care 3.
- From the Patient List, select Kelly Brady (Room 203).
- Click on **Go to Nurses' Station**.
- Click on **Chart** and then on **203**.
- Click on the **Consultations** tab and review the Psychiatric Consult.

5. According to information found in the Psychiatric Consult, Kelly Brady has major life events/precipitating stressors that are contributing to her depression. List several major stressors in Kelly Brady's life.

6. What behavioral symptoms is Kelly Brady experiencing related to depression?

7. Below, complete the intervention section of the treatment plan to address Kelly Brady's depression.

Area	Goal	Intervention
Environment/safety	Keep patient safe.	
Cognitive	Move patient beyond her preoccupation to other aspects of her life.	
Behavioral	Accomplish tasks and activities to counteract depression.	
Social skills	Provide experiences to counteract depression and social isolation and build self-esteem.	
Education	Educate patient about depression and the interventions and treatment that will be helpful.	

8. Explain how Kelly Brady's depression might be related to her pregnancy.

Kelly Brady's physician stated that he would recommend she take paroxetine after the birth of her baby. Complete the medication information below.

9. The trade name for paroxetine is _____, and the dose that was

   recommended was _____.

10. What is one clinical rationale for recommending paroxetine for Kelly Brady?

LESSON **8**

Anxiety Disorders

Reading Assignment: Anxiety-Related, Somatoform, and Dissociative Disorders (Chapter 30)

Patient: Dorothy Grant, Obstetrics Floor, Room 201

Goal: To care for a pregnant patient who is experiencing anxiety.

Objectives:

1. Identify characteristics of generalized anxiety disorder (GAD).
2. Describe physiologic responses to anxiety.
3. Define cognitive, behavioral, and affective responses to anxiety.
4. Identify stressors leading to a patient's anxiety.
5. List symptoms of acute stress disorder (ASD).
6. Know effective medications used to treat patients with anxiety.
7. Select treatment interventions and outcomes for a patient with anxiety.

Exercise 1

 Writing Activity

 30 minutes

1. In generalized anxiety disorder (GAD), the patient experiences the symptoms of anxiety both _____ and _____.

2. Indicate whether each of the following statements about GAD is true or false.

    a. _____ Family and twin studies suggest a genetic link to the development of GAD.

    b. _____ There might be a neurochemical dysregulation in GABA and other neurotransmitters.

    c. _____ Patients with GAD might have alterations in the number of benzodiazepine receptors.

    d. _____ Social and environmental factors do not play a role in the development of GAD.

    e. _____ There is no heredity involved in the development of GAD.

3. List at least five DSM-IV diagnoses consistent with anxiety-related disorders.

4. Specific nursing interventions are key in working with patients to reduce anxiety regardless of the diagnosis. List five of these key nursing interventions.

5. In working with patients with anxiety, the nurse's ultimate goal is to help patients develop

   _____

6. For patients with moderate to severe anxiety, medication may be a necessary intervention. In the table below, list the positive aspects and cautions associated with the use of antidepressant and anxiolytic medications in patients with anxiety.

Medication Class	Positive Aspects	Cautions
Antidepressant		
Anxiolytic		

Exercise 2

 Virtual Hospital Activity

 30 minutes

- Sign into work at Pacific View Regional Hospital on the Obstetrics Floor for Period of Care 2. (*Note:* If you are already in the virtual hospital from a previous exercise, click on **Leave the Floor** and then on **Restart the Program** to get to the sign-in window.)
- From the Patient List, select Dorothy Grant (Room 201).
- Click on **Get Report** and review the Clinical Report.
- Click on **Go to Nurses' Station** and then on **201** at the bottom of the screen.
- Click on **Patient Care** and then on **Nurse-Client Interactions**.
- Select and view the video titled **1115: Nurse-Patient Communication**. (*Note:* Check the virtual clock to see whether enough time has elapsed. You can use the fast-forward feature to advance the time by 2-minute intervals if the video is not yet available. Then click again on **Patient Care** and **Nurse-Client Interactions** to refresh the screen.)

1. One key nursing intervention to reduce anxiety is to encourage patients to discuss their feelings. What does the nurse say to encourage Dorothy Grant to discuss her situation? How does the nurse acknowledge her feelings?

2. The nurse assists Dorothy Grant in identifying priorities. She states that right now Dorothy Grant's first priority is her own _____ and _____.

3. Helping Dorothy Grant learn to use adaptive coping behaviors takes patience as well as an awareness that individuals learn and change at their own pace. What does the nurse say that indicates she has an understanding of this principle?

LESSON 8—ANXIETY DISORDERS 111

- Click on **Chart** and then on **201**.
- Click on the **Nursing Admission** and **History and Physical** tabs and review the information given.

  4. Acute stress disorder (ASD) results after exposure to a traumatic event that involves either the threat of death or injury to self or others or an actual injury to self or others. Was ASD one of the initial diagnoses for Dorothy Grant? Why or why not?

  5. Which of the following of Dorothy Grant's symptoms fit the DSM-IV-TR criteria for acute stress disorder (ASD)? Select all that apply.

   _____ Feelings of helplessness, fear, and shock

   _____ Distressing thoughts

   _____ Flashbacks

   _____ Amnesia

   _____ Sleep disturbance

   _____ Impairment in functioning socially

   _____ Decreased concentration

- Click on **Return to Room 201** and then on **MAR**.
- Click on tab **201**.
- Review the MAR to see if there are any medications ordered for Dorothy Grant's anxiety.

  6. Which of the following classifications of medications would typically be ordered for a patient with moderate to severe anxiety? Select all that apply.

   _____ Stimulants

   _____ Antidepressants

   _____ Antipsychotics

   _____ Antianxiety agents

Copyright © 2011, 2007 by Mosby, Inc., an affiliate of Elsevier Inc. All rights reserved.

7. Which of the following are important considerations in deciding whether or not to order medication to treat Dorothy Grant's anxiety? Select all that apply.

   _____ She is 30 weeks' pregnant and having possible contraindications.

   _____ Her anxiety is initially assessed to be at a moderate level.

   _____ Blunt force trauma to her abdomen may result in preterm delivery.

   _____ More time is needed to assess her anxiety level.

LESSON 9

Cognitive Disorders

Reading Assignment: Cognitive Disorders (Chapter 31)

Patient: Carlos Reyes, Skilled Nursing Floor, Room 504

Goal: To care for a patient who has symptoms of cardiovascular disease and also has a cognitive impairment.

Objectives:

1. Recognize the common disabilities in all cognitive disorders.
2. Compare and contrast characteristics of delirium and dementia.
3. Understand underlying principles of nursing interventions for patients with cognitive impairment.
4. Examine symptoms of severe disturbed behavior associated with dementia.
5. Identify nursing interventions used to care for a patient with agitation associated with dementia.
6. Describe successful nursing interventions used when caring for a patient with dementia.
7. Identify underlying medical conditions that can produce symptoms of delirium.
8. List medication used in the treatment of anxiety and agitation for a patient with dementia.
9. Provide practical strategies for families who will be caring for a family member with dementia.

Exercise 1

Writing Activity

30 minutes

1. A common thread in all cognitive disorders is the loss of the fundamental cognitive abilities of _____ and _____.

2. Distinguish between the cognitive disorders of delirium and dementia by matching each characteristic below with the disorder to which it applies.

Characteristic	Disorder
_____ Develops slowly over months and years	a. Delirium
_____ Involves multiple cognitive deficits, including impairment in memory without impairment in consciousness	b. Dementia
_____ Short-term memory impaired when assessed during a clear moment	
_____ Always secondary to another condition	
_____ Involves progressive deterioration	
_____ Acute onset; disturbance in consciousness and change in cognition develops over short period of time, usually hours to days but can last for months	
_____ Short-term memory lost initially; long-term memory fails slowly	
_____ May be reversible	
_____ Usually irreversible	

3. In addition to the usual symptoms of disorientation, confusion, memory loss, disorganized thinking, and poor judgment, secondary behavioral disturbances are common in individuals with dementia. These may include depression, hallucinations, delusions, agitation, insomnia, and wandering. Match each behavior type below with the corresponding example of how this type of behavior might manifest in an individual with dementia.

   Behavior Type

   _____ Aggressive psychomotor behavior

   _____ Nonaggressive psychomotor behavior

   _____ Verbally aggressive behavior

   _____ Passive behavior

   _____ Functionally impaired behavior

   _____ Other thought disorders

   Example of Manifestation

   a. Incontinence, poor hygiene

   b. Demanding, complaining, screaming, being disruptive

   c. Decreased activity, apathy, withdrawal, depression

   d. Hitting, kicking, pushing, scratching, being assaultive

   e. Restlessness, pacing, wandering

   f. Hallucinating, being delusional

4. Nursing interventions for cognitively impaired patients focus on which of the following?
   a. Protecting the patient's dignity
   b. Preserving functional status
   c. Promoting quality of life
   d. All of the above

5. Any major imbalance of body functions can disrupt cognitive functioning. Discuss how cardiac disorders and cardiac medications can be potential factors in a diagnosis of delirium.

6. Which of the following are symptoms that the nurse should look for in caring for a patient with delirium? Select all that apply.

   _____ Fluctuating level of consciousness

   _____ Slurred speech

   _____ Nonsensical thoughts

   _____ Day-night sleep reversal

   _____ Visual and/or tactile hallucinations

7. Planning care for a patient with dementia is geared toward the patient's _____ needs, because many cognitively impaired individuals live in the moment. The nurse who works with cognitively impaired patients must remember to smile and be pleasant, kind, and patient because the single most effective tool in caring for patients with dementia is the nurse's _____.

8. In providing care for patients with dementia, priority is given to nursing interventions that maintain the patient's optimal level of functioning. With that in mind, complete the table below and on the next page by identifying effective nursing interventions for each component of care listed.

Component of Care	Interventions
Communication	
Scheduling	
Orientation and memory aids	
Toileting	

Component of Care	Interventions
Nutrition	
Wandering	
Medication	
Agitation	
Family and community	

Exercise 2

 Virtual Hospital Activity

 30 minutes

- Sign in to work at Pacific View Regional Hospital on the Skilled Nursing Floor for Period of Care 2. (*Note:* If you are already in the virtual hospital from a previous exercise, click on **Leave the Floor** and then on **Restart the Program** to get to the sign-in window.)
- From the Patient List, select Carlos Reyes (Room 504).
- Click on **Get Report** and read the Clinical Report.

1. As noted in the change-of-shift report, what have been Carlos Reyes' most problematic symptoms?

- Click on **Go to Nurses' Station** and then on **504** at the bottom of the screen.
- Click on **Patient Care** and then on **Nurse-Client Interactions**.
- Select and view the video titled **1120: The Agitated Patient**. (*Note:* Check the virtual clock to see whether enough time has elapsed. You can use the fast-forward feature to advance the time by 2-minute intervals if the video is not yet available. Then click again on **Patient Care** and **Nurse-Client Interactions** to refresh the screen.)

2. Which of the following intervention(s) did the nurse use to respond to Carlos Reyes' agitation? Select all that apply.

   _____ Ignored the difficult behavior

   _____ Listened to the patient and the patient's daughter

   _____ Spoke in a calm, reassuring manner to decrease stress in the environment

   _____ Modified the original plan to meet the patient's needs

LESSON 9—COGNITIVE DISORDERS 119

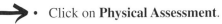
- Click on **Physical Assessment**.
- Click on **Head and Neck** and then on **Mental Status** and review the assessment.

3. What symptoms in the mental status assessment indicate that Carlos Reyes is experiencing cognitive impairments?

4. Which of the following symptoms associated with aggression (sometimes seen in patients with cognitive impairments) is Carlos Reyes exhibiting? Select all that apply.

   _____ Extreme anxiety

   _____ Irritability

   _____ Soft-spoken

   _____ Confusion

   _____ Memory intact

   _____ Disorientation

- Click on **Patient Care** and then on **Nurse-Client Interactions**.
- Select and view the video titled **1140: Assessing for Referrals**. (*Note:* Check the virtual clock to see whether enough time has elapsed. You can use the fast-forward feature to advance the time by 2-minute intervals if the video is not yet available. Then click again on **Patient Care** and **Nurse-Client Interactions** to refresh the screen.)

5. Assess the son's understanding of Carlos Reyes' illness. What action should the nurse take after her brief interaction with the son?

Copyright © 2011, 2007 by Mosby, Inc., an affiliate of Elsevier Inc. All rights reserved.

120 VIRTUAL CLINICAL EXCURSIONS FOR PSYCHIATRIC NURSING

Exercise 3

Virtual Hospital Activity

45 minutes

- Sign in to work at Pacific View Regional Hospital on the Skilled Nursing Floor for Period of Care 3. (*Note:* If you are already in the virtual hospital from a previous exercise, click on **Leave the Floor** and then on **Restart the Program** to get to the sign-in window.)
- From the Patient List, select Carlos Reyes (Room 504).
- Click on **Go to Nurses' Station**.
- Click on **Chart** and then on **504**.
- Click on the **History and Physical** and **Nursing Admission** tabs and review the information given.

  1. Which of the following factors may be contributing to Carlos Reyes' confusion? Select all that apply.

     _____ Change in environment

     _____ Recent myocardial infarction

     _____ History of dementia

     _____ Medication regimen

  2. If Carlos Reyes returns to his daughter's home after discharge, discuss the problems that his daughter may have in caring for him.

- Click on **Return to Nurses' Station** and then on **504** at the bottom of the screen.
- Click on **Patient Care** and then on **Nurse-Client Interactions**.
- Select and view the video titled **1500: The Confused Patient**. (*Note:* Check the virtual clock to see whether enough time has elapsed. You can use the fast-forward feature to advance the time by 2-minute intervals if the video is not yet available. Then click again on **Patient Care** and **Nurse-Client Interactions** to refresh the screen.)

Copyright © 2011, 2007 by Mosby, Inc., an affiliate of Elsevier Inc. All rights reserved.

LESSON 9—COGNITIVE DISORDERS 121

3. Describe the approach the nurse used in dealing with Carlos Reyes' confusion.

- Click on **Patient Care** and then on **Nurse-Client Interactions**.
- Select and view the video titled **1505: Family Teaching—Dementia**. (*Note:* Check the virtual clock to see whether enough time has elapsed. You can use the fast-forward feature to advance the time by 2-minute intervals if the video is not yet available. Then click again on **Patient Care** and **Nurse-Client Interactions** to refresh the screen.)

4. Interventions that involve family members of patients with dementia are critical to the success of the discharge plan. In the interaction with Carlos Reyes' daughter, what interventions did the nurse use?

- Click on **MAR** and then on **504**.
- Identify the medication ordered for anxiety and agitation.
- Click on **Return to Room 504**.
- Click on the **Drug** icon in the lower left corner of the screen.
- Review the information for the medication identified in the MAR.

5. Based on your review of the Drug Guide, provide the information requested below for the drug ordered for Carlos Reyes' anxiety and agitation.

Generic name of medication

Chemical classification

Mechanism of action

Therapeutic effect

Indication

Dosage

Side effects

Nursing indications

- Click on **Return to Room 504**.
- Click on **Patient Care** and then on **Nurse-Client Interactions**.
- Select and view the video titled **1525: Family Conflict—Discharge Plan**. (*Note:* Check the virtual clock to see whether enough time has elapsed. You can use the fast-forward feature to advance the time by 2-minute intervals if the video is not yet available. Then click again on **Patient Care** and **Nurse-Client Interactions** to refresh the screen.)
- Click on **Chart** and then on **504**.
- Click on the **Consultations** tab and review the Discharge Coordinator Consult.

6. Describe the family conflict about Carlos Reyes' care and its significance in planning for discharge. Describe how the nurse should approach the family situation.

7. Support for Carlos Reyes' family members will be crucial to help them in their caretaking role. Given Carlos Reyes' illness and family situation, what types of community support might be beneficial?

8. Practical recommendations for discharge are necessary for caregivers who must care for family members with dementia, especially those who are also agitated and demonstrate aggressive behavior. Using what you know about Carlos Reyes, provide some practical approaches that you would recommend to his daughter in each of the areas listed below.

Area of Focus	Practical Approaches
Environment	
Communication	
Self-care basics	

LESSON 10

Substance-Related Disorders

Reading Assignment: Substance-Related Disorders (Chapter 34)

Patient: Laura Wilson, Obstetrics Floor, Room 206

Goal: To care for a patient with acute medical needs who also has a diagnosis of polysubstance abuse.

Objectives:

1. Discuss the prevalence of drug use in the United States.
2. Understand terms used to describe patients who have substance-related disorders.
3. Identify risks associated with drug use and pregnancy.
4. Identify precipitating stressors, coping mechanisms, and resources of a patient with polysubstance abuse.
5. Describe the elements included in the assessment of a patient with polysubstance abuse.
6. Identify key aspects of the treatment plan to include in the teaching for a patient with polysubstance abuse.
7. Understand the importance of relapse prevention for a patient with a diagnosis of substance abuse.
8. Describe critical elements of discharge planning for a patient who has abused substances.

Exercise 1

 Writing Activity

 30 minutes

1. Substance abuse disorders among the general population are one of the most significant health issues of our time. Which of the following statements regarding substance use are correct? Select all that apply.

   _____ 20 million Americans over the age of 12 use illicit drugs.

   _____ Marijuana is the most widely used illegal drug in the United States.

   _____ Alcohol abuse is the primary drug problem in North America and ranks as one of the leading causes of death and disability in the United States.

   _____ In 1999, the U.S. Surgeon General estimated that one-third to one-half of all patients undergoing psychiatric treatment abuse alcohol or drugs.

   _____ Cocaine and its derivatives were used by almost 1.9 million Americans in 2008.

2. Not everyone who uses drugs becomes an abuser; however, for some individuals, drug use begins with _____ use, which progresses to frequent use, and eventually leads to _____ and _____.

3. When the nurse is discussing drug use, it is important to understand certain terminology related to abuse. Match each of the terms below with its definition.

Term	Definition
_____ Dependence	a. Occurs when the dependent person does not recognize the destructive nature of alcohol and other drug (AOD) use
_____ Abuse	
_____ Denial	b. Occurs when there is coexistence of substance abuse and a psychiatric disorder in a patient
_____ Dual diagnosis	
_____ Physical dependence	c. Leads to a substance-specific syndrome causing clinically significant distress or impairment
_____ Withdrawal	d. Marked by the physiologic need for increasing amounts of the substance despite trying to cut down, along with continued use of the substance even when physical, social, and emotional processes are compromised; has replaced the term *addiction*
_____ Tolerance	

e. A maladaptive pattern of substance use leading to clinically significant impairment or distress

f. Results from a biologic need that occurs when the body becomes used to having the substance in the system

g. Occurs when continued use results in more of the substance being needed to produce the same effect

4. In addition to taking a history and performing a physical examination, the assessment process for drug use includes laboratory testing. Discuss the importance of drug toxicology testing of patients who present with symptoms of possible substance abuse.

5. Which of the following are possible signs and symptoms of a substance-related disorder? Select all that apply.

   _____ Drowsiness

   _____ Flushed face

   _____ Clean and neat appearance

   _____ Organized thoughts

   _____ Slurred speech

   _____ Tremors

   _____ Watery or reddened eyes

6. The assessment of a patient with polysubstance abuse must be comprehensive and include several key categories. List the most important areas you believe should be included in the assessment and one question that the nurse might ask within each of these areas.

Exercise 2

 Virtual Hospital Activity

 30 minutes

- Sign in to work at Pacific View Regional Hospital on the Obstetrics Floor for Period of Care 1. (*Note:* If you are already in the virtual hospital from a previous exercise, click on **Leave the Floor** and then on **Restart the Program** to get to the sign-in window.)
- From the Patient List, select Laura Wilson (Room 206).
- Click on **Get Report** and read the Clinical Report.
- Click on **Go to Nurses' Station**.
- Click on **Chart** and then on **206**.
- Click on the **Emergency Department** tab and review the record.

1. Which of the following pieces of information would indicate that Laura Wilson may be abusing drugs? Select all that apply.

    _____ Found unconscious

    _____ Nausea and diarrhea

    _____ HIV-positive

    _____ History of drug abuse

2. The assessment of chemical impairment is complex because the simultaneous use of many substances (polydrug abuse) is becoming more common. Laura Wilson's urine drug toxicology screen came back positive for cocaine and marijuana. Complete the table below and on the next page regarding the characteristics of these two drugs.

Substance	Route	Signs and Symptoms of Use	Withdrawal Signs and Symptoms	Consequences of Use
Cocaine				

130 VIRTUAL CLINICAL EXCURSIONS FOR PSYCHIATRIC NURSING

Substance	Route	Signs and Symptoms of Use	Withdrawal Signs and Symptoms	Consequences of Use
Marijuana				

- Click on the **Nursing Admission** tab and review the information given.

3. In addition to crack cocaine, marijuana, and caffeine, there are two other drugs Laura Wilson is abusing. The report indicates these drugs are _____ and _____.

4. No drug can be considered safe when used by a woman during pregnancy. In the table below and on the next page, list the potential effects on a fetus associated with each substance that Laura Wilson has abused.

Substance	Effect(s) on Fetus
Nicotine	
Marijuana	

Copyright © 2011, 2007 by Mosby, Inc., an affiliate of Elsevier Inc. All rights reserved.

Substance	Effect(s) on Fetus
Opioids	
Alcohol	

5. The Nursing Admission record contains information regarding Laura Wilson's precipitating stressors. Which of the following are stressors that Laura Wilson has identified? Select all that apply.

   _____ Parents disapprove of her lifestyle

   _____ HIV-positive status

   _____ Unplanned pregnancy

   _____ Need to quit "crack"

   _____ Boyfriend out of town

6. Which of the following is the best coping resource available to Laura Wilson at this time?
   a. Younger sister
   b. Boyfriend
   c. Parents
   d. Roommate

7. Laura Wilson's most frequently used coping mechanisms up to this point have been

   _____ and _____.

132 Virtual Clinical Excursions for Psychiatric Nursing

Exercise 3

 Virtual Hospital Activity

 30 minutes

- Sign in to work at Pacific View Regional Hospital on the Obstetrics Floor for Period of Care 2. (*Note:* If you are already in the virtual hospital from a previous exercise, click on **Leave the Floor** and then on **Restart the Program** to get to the sign-in window.)
- From the Patient List, select Laura Wilson (Room 206).
- Click on **Go to Nurses' Station** and then on **206** at the bottom of the screen.
- Click on **Patient Care** and then on **Nurse-Client Interactions**.
- Select and view the video titled **1115: Teaching—Effects of Drug Use**. (*Note:* Check the virtual clock to see whether enough time has elapsed. You can use the fast-forward feature to advance the time by 2-minute intervals if the video is not yet available. Then click again on **Patient Care** and **Nurse-Client Interactions** to refresh the screen.)

1. Which of the following statements made by Laura Wilson during the interaction with the nurse best illustrate(s) her lack of understanding regarding substance abuse? Select all that apply.

    _____ "The baby will help me stay on track."

    _____ "It's not like I'm addicted. I can quit anytime."

    _____ "It's not like the baby will be addicted."

    _____ "I have quit for a month or two."

2. Which of the following statements made by Laura Wilson during the interaction with the nurse indicate(s) that Laura Wilson might be ready to abstain from drugs? Select all that apply.

    _____ "It wasn't a hard decision for me. I am looking forward to this baby."

    _____ "I can go for a while without taking drugs."

    _____ "My mom doesn't believe I can do it."

    _____ "I'll do whatever it takes to keep my baby."

3. What do you see as the barriers to Laura Wilson's abstinence from drugs?

Copyright © 2011, 2007 by Mosby, Inc., an affiliate of Elsevier Inc. All rights reserved.

LESSON 10—SUBSTANCE-RELATED DISORDERS   133

4. Evaluate the nurse's role in educating Laura Wilson on the effects of drug use.

→ • Click on **MAR** and then on **206**.
   • Locate the medication prescribed for Laura Wilson for pain.
   • Click on **Return to Room 206**.
   • Click on the **Drug** icon in the lower left corner of the screen and review the medication identified in the MAR.

5. The medication ordered for Laura Wilson's pain is _____. In Laura Wilson's situation, the two most important features of this medication are that it is safe to

   use during _____ and that it is not _____.

6. An important aspect of Laura Wilson's treatment plan will be the teaching plan. Below, match each of Laura Wilson's education needs with the resource you think would be most helpful in providing/reinforcing this teaching.

   Education Need   **Resource**

   _____ Understanding her HIV-positive   a. Well-baby clinic and parental support
         status
                                                b. Community-based self-help group and
   _____ Caring for her newborn   individual motivational and cognitive
                                                   behavioral approaches
   _____ Drug abstinence
                                                c. HIV counselor/HIV clinic
   _____ Handling family conflict
                                                d. Hospital social worker/discharge planner
   _____ Community resources
                                                e. Family counseling

7. Relapses are common during a person's recovery. For patients who abuse substances, an important aspect of discharge planning is relapse prevention. The goal for relapse prevention is to help the person learn from these situations so that periods of

   _____ can be lengthened over time.

Copyright © 2011, 2007 by Mosby, Inc., an affiliate of Elsevier Inc. All rights reserved.

134 VIRTUAL CLINICAL EXCURSIONS FOR PSYCHIATRIC NURSING

8. Relapse should not be viewed as a total failure, but rather as an opportunity for a renewed and refined effort toward change. Discuss relapse prevention strategies you think the nurse should include in working with Laura Wilson.

9. Community resources will be needed to assist Laura Wilson in her recovery. Which of the following community resources might be helpful to her?
   a. 12-step recovery program
   b. Intensive outpatient program
   c. Relapse prevention group
   d. Individual, group, or family therapy
   e. All of the above

LESSON 11

Eating Disorders

Reading Assignment: Eating Disorders (Chapter 36)

Patient: Tiffany Sheldon, Pediatrics Floor, Room 305

Goal: To provide nursing care for a patient with an eating disorder who also has comorbid psychiatric symptoms.

Objectives:

1. Discuss prevalence of eating disorders.
2. Identify types of eating disorders and their associated symptoms.
3. Identify predisposing factors and precipitating stressors related to eating disorders.
4. Assess interactions between nurses and a patient with an eating disorder.
5. Identify coping resources and coping mechanisms related to eating disorders.
6. Apply the nursing process in caring for a patient with an eating disorder.
7. List the primary goals in the management of a patient with anorexia.
8. Develop a treatment plan for a patient with an eating disorder.

Exercise 1

 Writing Activity

 30 minutes

1. Indicate whether each of the following statements is true or false.

    a. _____ Anorexia nervosa and bulimia nervosa are the only specific eating disorder diagnoses outlined in the Diagnostic and Statistical Manual (DSM-IV-TR).

    b. _____ Anorexia affects up to 3.7% of women during their lifetime.

    c. _____ Approximately 90% of patients with eating disorders are female.

    d. _____ 50% of dieters progress to pathologic dieting.

    e. _____ The AXIS I diagnoses most closely associated with eating disorders are mood disorders, anxiety, dissociative disorders, and substance abuse.

    f. _____ The onset of bulimia nervosa is between 15 and 24 years of age.

    g. _____ The causes of eating disorders are multifactorial.

    h. _____ A history of sexual abuse is less common in those with eating disorders than in the general population.

2. Symptoms are reflective of the type of eating disorder; however, there are symptoms common to both anorexia and bulimia. Which of the following symptoms are common to both of these eating disorders? Select all that apply.

    _____ Extreme concern about appearance

    _____ Skipping meals occasionally

    _____ Restrictions intake at times

    _____ Overexercising

    _____ Overeating under stress

    _____ Purging through vomiting, laxatives, or diuretics

    _____ Bingeing or overeating at times

    _____ Perceiving oneself as fat even though underweight

    _____ Comfortable in social settings especially with the opposite sex

    _____ Perfectionist traits

3. Disordered eating can lead to serious medical complications. Which of the following can result from an eating disorder?
   a. Dehydration, hypokalemia, metabolic alkalosis, and acidosis
   b. Hypotension, bradycardia, and hypothermia
   c. Hypoglycemia, menstrual dysfunction, and reflex constipation
   d. Esophagitis, dental enamel erosion, and enlarged salivary and parotid glands
   e. Cardiac arrhythmias and cardiomyopathy
   f. All of the above

4. How do sociocultural factors regarding body size affect the prevalence of eating disorders in adolescent females?

5. Numerous psychologic factors can predispose a person to develop an eating disorder. Which of the following personality characteristics are associated with eating disorders? Select all that apply.

   _____ Perfectionism exhibited by rigid, meticulous, ritualistic, obsessive-compulsive behaviors

   _____ Ambivalent feelings of self-esteem; belief that worth is solely based on appearance

   _____ Persuasive sense of ineffectiveness and helplessness; no control over life

   _____ Difficulty expressing emotions; rapidly fluctuating moods

   _____ Interpersonal distrust due to pain in their lives stemming from abuse, neglect, trauma

   _____ Inability to correctly identify and respond to bodily sensations

   _____ Mature and compliant

6. Comorbid psychiatric illnesses are prevalent in patients with eating disorders. Complete the table below by providing examples of psychiatric illnesses that often accompany each of the eating disorders.

Eating Disorder	Common Psychiatric Comorbidity Examples
Anorexia nervosa	
Bulimia nervosa	

7. Discuss the family characteristics that may predispose an individual to an eating disorder.

8. What sociocultural biases do you have regarding individuals with eating disorders that result in them being severely underweight or overweight?

LESSON 11—EATING DISORDERS 139

Exercise 2

 Virtual Hospital Activity

 15 minutes

- Sign in to work at Pacific View Regional Hospital on the Pediatrics Floor for Period of Care 1. (*Note:* If you are already in the virtual hospital from a previous exercise, click on **Leave the Floor** and then on **Restart the Program** to get to the sign-in window.)
- From the Patient List, select Tiffany Sheldon (Room 305).
- Click on **Get Report** and read the Clinical Report.
- Click on **Go to Nurses' Station** and then on **305** at the bottom of the screen.
- Read the **Initial Observations**.

1. What behaviors is Tiffany Sheldon exhibiting that may be indicative of comorbid psychiatric disorders?

- Click on **Patient Care** and then on **Head and Neck**.
- Click on **Mental Status** and review the assessment data.

2. Which of the following characteristics in the mental status assessment coincide with the change-of-shift report and Initial Observations? Select all that apply.

   _____ Good eye contact

   _____ Listless

   _____ Flat affect

   _____ Energetic

   _____ Avoids eye contact

   _____ Withdrawn

Copyright © 2011, 2007 by Mosby, Inc., an affiliate of Elsevier Inc. All rights reserved.

- Click on **Patient Care** and then on **Nurse-Client Interactions**.
- Select and view the video titled **0730: Initial Assessment**. (*Note:* Check the virtual clock to see whether enough time has elapsed. You can use the fast-forward feature to advance the time by 2-minute intervals if the video is not yet available. Then click again on **Patient Care** and **Nurse-Client Interactions** to refresh the screen.)

3. How would you characterize Tiffany Sheldon's responses to the nurse who is caring for her?

- Click on **Chart** and then on **305**.
- Click on the **Physician's Orders** tab and review the information given.

4. What orders are written that indicate multidisciplinary assessments being implemented for Tiffany Sheldon's care?

- Click on the **History and Physical** tab and review the information given.

5. Tiffany Sheldon's medical diagnoses are _____, _____, and _____.

- Click on the **Nursing Admission** tab and review the information given.

6. List at least two possible predisposing psychologic and family environmental factors associated with Tiffany Sheldon's eating disorder.

LESSON 11—EATING DISORDERS 141

Exercise 3

 Virtual Hospital Activity

 30 minutes

- Sign in to work at Pacific View Regional Hospital on the Pediatrics Floor for Period of Care 3. (*Note:* If you are already in the virtual hospital from a previous exercise, click on **Leave the Floor** and then on **Restart the Program** to get to the sign-in window.)
- From the Patient List, select Tiffany Sheldon (Room 305).
- Click on **Go to Nurses' Station** and then on **305** at the bottom of the screen.
- Click on **Patient Care** and then on **Nurse-Client Interactions**.
- Select and view the video titled **1500: Relapse—Contributing Factors**. (*Note:* Check the virtual clock to see whether enough time has elapsed. You can use the fast-forward feature to advance the time by 2-minute intervals if the video is not yet available. Then click again on **Patient Care** and **Nurse-Client Interactions** to refresh the screen.)

1. Tiffany Sheldon's predisposing factors make her especially vulnerable to environmental pressures and stress. Which stressors have contributed to the current relapse of her eating disorder? Select all that apply.

   _____ Parents were divorced 3 years ago.

   _____ Family does not understand her problem.

   _____ Mom is angry and "disgusted."

   _____ She visited her father in Florida 2 weeks ago.

- Click on **Chart** and then on **305**.
- Click on the **Mental Health** tab and read the Psychiatric/Mental Health Assessment.

2. Characteristic of a patient with anorexia, Tiffany Sheldon's main unhealthy coping

   mechanism is _____.

3. For people with anorexia, the issue is not really about their weight, but rather about controlling their life and fears. Tiffany Sheldon's statement,

   "_____" is an example
   of this overriding concern.

4. In addition to Tiffany Sheldon's nursing diagnosis of Imbalanced nutrition less than body requirements, identify two nursing diagnoses that best describe the psychologic components to her eating disorder.

Copyright © 2011, 2007 by Mosby, Inc., an affiliate of Elsevier Inc. All rights reserved.

142 Virtual Clinical Excursions for Psychiatric Nursing

- Click on **Return to Room 305**.
- Click on **Patient Care** and then on **Nurse-Client Interactions**.
- Select and view the video titled **1530: Facilitating Success**. (*Note:* Check the virtual clock to see whether enough time has elapsed. You can use the fast-forward feature to advance the time by 2-minute intervals if the video is not yet available. Then click again on **Patient Care** and **Nurse-Client Interactions** to refresh the screen.)

5. For a patient to be able to recover from an eating disorder, one of the most important aspects is motivation to change the behavior. What statement does Tiffany Sheldon make that would best define her motivation level? Discuss the impact her motivational level will have in preventing relapse.

6. Therapeutic management of symptoms associated with an eating disorder will typically follow a sequence starting with interventions designed to deal with the immediate crisis followed by those of a psychotherapeutic nature designed to help deal more effectively with the disorder. Place the three objectives below in order of their priority in the management of Tiffany Sheldon's anorexia.

Objective	Order of Priority
_____ Increase her self-esteem so she does not feel the need to attain perfection, which she equates with thinness	a. First
	b. Second
_____ Help her reestablish appropriate eating behavior	c. Third
_____ Increase weight to at least 90% of her average body weight for her height	

- Click on **Chart** and then on **305**.
- Click on the **Consultations** tab and review the Psychiatric Consult.

7. Tiffany Sheldon has two simultaneous plans of care being implemented. One plan involves the eating contract, and the other is the plan devised as a result of the psychiatric consult. Complete the table below by identifying interventions planned for the various elements of the psychosocial treatment plan.

Element of the Psychosocial Treatment Plan	Specific Interventions
Individual therapy	
Family conference/ family therapy	
Relationship to eating contract	
Medication	

LESSON 12

Nutraceuticals and Mental Health

 Reading Assignment: Nutraceuticals and Mental Health (Chapter 38)

Patient: Kelly Brady, Obstetrics Floor, Room 203

Goal: To provide nursing care to a patient with anxiety and depression utilizing alternative and complementary therapies.

Objectives:

1. Define *nutraceuticals*.
2. Define *alternative therapies*.
3. Compare and contrast conventional medicine and alternative therapies.
4. Discuss the trend toward the use of alternative therapies.
5. List the types of alternative therapies.
6. Refer patients to reliable resources on alternative therapies.
7. Discuss alternative therapies for a patient with depression and anxiety.

Exercise 1

 Writing Activity

 30 minutes

1. The biomedical and holistic models of health care are based on different assumptions. Match each of the assumptions below to the correct health care model.

Assumption	Model
_____ The focus of health care is on strengthening one's inner resistance to disease.	a. Biomedical
_____ Health care is based on the scientific method of identifying causes of disease and implementing curative treatments to correct aberrant physiology.	b. Holistic
_____ Health can be achieved by "healing from within" or enhancing one's innate healing powers.	
_____ Infections are defined by the germ theory.	
_____ Illness prevention is based on proper hygiene, public sanitation, and personal lifestyle choices.	

2. _____ therapy refers to a broad range of healing philosophies and approaches that traditional medicine does not commonly use, accept, understand, or make available. _____ therapy refers to those used in conjunction with conventional therapies. Together, these are called _____, or referred to as CAM for short. _____ refers to herbal medicines and dietary supplements.

3. It is important for the nurse to become familiar with the nontraditional therapies mentioned above. Which of the following statements are reasons that this may be important in nursing care? Select all that apply.

   _____ 80% of the world's population relies on alternative therapies.

   _____ The FDA does not regulate herbal remedies and supplements.

   _____ One in three consumers in the United States uses alternative therapies.

   _____ Some people think herbal treatments that are labeled as "natural" are harmless.

   _____ Of the people who use alternative therapies with traditional medicine, less than 50% tell their conventional practitioners.

   _____ Some alternative therapies interfere with traditional treatments.

4. American consumers are increasingly choosing to use alternative therapies in conjunction with conventional therapies. Why do you think this is?

5. In thinking about the reasons more people are turning to complementary and alternative therapies, what steps do you think the nurse could take to demonstrate his or her willingness to work closely with patients who may also be using CAM?

6. The nurse must be able to direct patients to reliable and professional information on complementary and alternative therapies. One organization that disseminates information on CAM to practitioners and the public is the National Center for Complementary and Alternative Medicine (NCCAM), a branch of the National Institutes of Health (NIH). According to the NCCAM, complementary and alternative health practices are grouped into categories. Provide at least one example of a complementary or alternative therapy and/or treatment for each of the categories listed below.

Category	Examples
Whole medical	
Mind-body	
Nutraceutical	

Exercise 2

 Virtual Hospital Activity

 30 minutes

- Sign in to work at Pacific View Regional Hospital on the Obstetrics Floor for Period of Care 3. (*Note:* If you are already in the virtual hospital from a previous exercise, click on **Leave the Floor** and then on **Restart the Program** to get to the sign-in window.)
- From the Patient List, select Kelly Brady (Room 203).
- Click on **Go to Nurses' Station**.
- Click on **Chart** and then on **203**.
- Click on the **Nursing Admission** tab and review the information given.

1. Two questions in the Nursing Admission refer to Kelly Brady's use of complementary/alternative therapies and to her spiritual and cultural practices. What are these two questions, and how did Kelly Brady answer them?

2. According to Kelly Brady's Nursing Admission, she reads the Bible and prays and has arranged for her pastor to visit her in the hospital. Discuss the benefits of prayer as a CAM therapy.

→ • Click on the **Consultations** tab and review the Psychiatric Consult.

3. Which of the following stressors apply specifically to Kelly Brady?
    a. Her mother has been diagnosed with cancer, and her parents are out of town for treatment.
    b. Her husband's job is not stable, but they are moving to a more expensive home.
    c. She has a high stress job, and her work performance has been declining.
    d. She and her baby are facing potential health problems due to preeclampsia and probable premature delivery.
    e. All of the above.

4. Kelly Brady has multiple stressors in her life that are creating anxiety and depression. Which of the following conventional treatments have been recommended to alleviate her anxiety and depression? Select all that apply.

    _____ Paroxetine 20 mg, postcesarean section

    _____ Cognitive, couples, and family therapies

    _____ Education regarding depression

    _____ Anxiety-reduction techniques

→ • Click the **Mental Health** tab and review the Psychiatric/Mental Health Assessment.

5. What coping methods has Kelly Brady been using to cope with her stress? (*Hint:* See page 5 of the Psychiatric/Mental Health Assessment.)

6. Has Kelly Brady used any alternative therapies in the past?

7. There are several integrative approaches to the treatment of anxiety and depression. List several approaches that you believe might be beneficial in treating both anxiety and depression. Which of these approaches are found in Kelly Brady's treatment plan?

8. Based on what you know about Kelly Brady's past attempts to control her anxiety and depression, what other alternative treatments or therapies would you recommend for her?

LESSON 13

Survivors of Violence and Trauma

Reading Assignment: Survivors of Violence and Trauma (Chapter 39)

Patient: Dorothy Grant, Obstetrics Floor, Room 201

Goal: To care for a patient who is a victim of domestic violence.

Objectives:

1. Define *domestic violence* (also called *partner abuse*).
2. Understand difference between myths and realities associated with survivors of abuse.
3. Describe the stages in the cycle of violence and explain the role it plays in partner abuse.
4. Identify strengths and coping strategies of a female patient who is experiencing abuse or violence.
5. Discuss the nursing assessment and interventions for a patient experiencing domestic violence.
6. Identify characteristics of violent families.
7. Recognize characteristics of a woman who is a victim of partner abuse.
8. Understand common barriers that prevent battered spouses from leaving the abusive relationship.
9. Describe critical elements of discharge planning for a patient who is being abused.

154 VIRTUAL CLINICAL EXCURSIONS FOR PSYCHIATRIC NURSING

Exercise 1

 Writing Activity

 15 minutes

1. Define *partner abuse* (or *domestic violence*).

2. Violent behaviors associated with partner abuse can include isolation, threats, and

   _____, as well as physical, sexual, psychologic, emotional, and

   economic _____. Underlying these behaviors is the desire for

   _____ and _____.

3. There are several myths regarding victims of partner abuse. Match each myth below with the reality.

Myth	Reality
_____ Abused spouses can end the violence by leaving their abuser.	a. Battering often begins or escalates during pregnancy. Prior partner abuse increases the risk for abuse during pregnancy.
_____ The victim can learn to stop doing things that provoke the violence.	b. In a battering relationship, the abuser does not need a provocation. It is a pattern of behavior by the abuser; it is not about the behavior of the victim.
_____ Being pregnant protects a woman from battering.	c. Many women reveal their situation to friends and family, but often they are met with denial and disbelief, discouraging them from further disclosing.
_____ Abused women quietly accept the abuse by trying to conceal it, not reporting it, or failing to seek help.	d. Separation can bring on an increase in harassment and violence. A woman is in greatest danger when she attempts to leave a controlling mate.

Copyright © 2011, 2007 by Mosby, Inc., an affiliate of Elsevier Inc. All rights reserved.

4. One accepted view of why women endure partner abuse is referred to as the "cycle of violence." Describe the three stages of the cycle of violence and give an example of the woman's thoughts and feelings in each of the three stages to help explain this phenomenon.

5. What are your personal thoughts about domestic violence?

156 VIRTUAL CLINICAL EXCURSIONS FOR PSYCHIATRIC NURSING

Exercise 2

Virtual Hospital Activity

 30 minutes

- Sign in to work at Pacific View Regional Hospital on the Obstetrics Floor for Period of Care 2. (*Note:* If you are already in the virtual hospital from a previous exercise, click on **Leave the Floor** and then on **Restart the Program** to get to the sign-in window.)
- From the Patient List, select Dorothy Grant (Room 201).
- Click on **Go to Nurses' Station**.
- Click on **Chart** and then on **201**.
- Click on and review the **Nursing Admission**, **Mental Health**, and **Consultations** tabs.

1. Which of the following forms of abuse is Dorothy Grant experiencing? Select all that apply.

    _____ Physical

    _____ Sexual

    _____ Emotional

    _____ Neglect

    _____ Economic

2. Dorothy Grant is a member of one of the special populations that are vulnerable to abuse. These include children, older adults, and the developmentally disabled, as well as the

    _____ partner. The most widespread form of family violence is abuse of

    _____ partners.

3. Several general characteristics are common in families that experience violence. These characteristics are listed in the left column below. In the right column, identify any specific characteristics of Dorothy Grant's family that correspond to these general characteristics.

General Characteristics of Families That Experience Violence	**Characteristics of Dorothy Grant's Family**
Multigenerational history of violence	
Social isolation	
Use and abuse of power	
Alcohol and drug abuse	

4. What are Dorothy Grant's strengths in dealing with her abusive situation?

5. What are Dorothy Grant's coping strategies in dealing with her abusive relationship?

6. Depression is a common response of women in abusive relationships. According to Dorothy Grant's depression scale, her level of depression is _____.

Exercise 3

 Virtual Hospital Activity

 45 minutes

- Sign in to work at Pacific View Regional Hospital on the Obstetrics Floor for Period of Care 2. (*Note:* If you are already in the virtual hospital from a previous exercise, click on **Leave the Floor** and then on **Restart the Program** to get to the sign-in window.)
- From the Patient List, select Dorothy Grant (Room 201).
- Click on **Go to Nurses' Station** and then on **201** at the bottom of the screen.
- Click on **Patient Care** and then on **Nurse-Client Interactions**.
- Select and view the video titled **1115: Nurse-Patient Communication**. (*Note:* Check the virtual clock to see whether enough time has elapsed. You can use the fast-forward feature to advance the time by 2-minute intervals if the video is not yet available. Then click again on **Patient Care** and **Nurse-Client Interactions** to refresh the screen.)

1. The primary goal of intervention is empowerment, which is found to be very effective in working with battered women. In the video interaction, the nurse uses various techniques that support this goal when interacting with Dorothy Grant. Below and on the next page, cite specific examples that illustrate how the nurse is applying each of the listed principles associated with empowerment. (*Hint:* If you are unable to find an example from the nurse's responses, create a response that the nurse could make to meet the empowerment goal.)

Principles Associated with Empowerment	Nurse's Response
Mutual sharing of knowledge and information	
Nurse strategizing with the abuse survivor	

Principles Associated with Empowerment	Nurse's Response
Helping the abuse survivor to recognize societal influences	
Respecting abuse survivor's competence and experiences	

2. The nurse uses other therapeutic responses when interacting with Dorothy Grant. Match each therapeutic technique listed below with the corresponding response by the nurse.

Technique	Nurse's Response
_____ Mutual goal sharing	a. "Feeling scared is a perfectly normal reaction."
_____ Focusing	b. "The nurse specialist and the social worker work together to identify your immediate needs."
_____ Using broad open-ended questions	
_____ Listening	c. "Right now, your first priority is your well-being and the well-being of your baby."
	d. "Would you like to talk about your concerns now?" and "Is there anything I can do to help?"

3. The immediate goal of the nurse in working with Dorothy Grant is to develop trust. In order to develop trust, the nurse must express nonjudgmental listening and psychologic support. Do you think the nurse accomplished this in the video? Why or why not?

4. Which of the following are constraints that will make it difficult for Dorothy Grant to leave her husband? Select all that apply.

   _____ She is still in love with her husband.

   _____ She lacks housing and financial resources.

   _____ Her church affiliation supports marriage.

   _____ The societal stigma attached to abuse and divorce.

   _____ Domestic violence reporting is not mandatory in any state.

   _____ Her husband is in jail.

5. Dorothy Grant has left her husband twice before and returned. For a woman who is experiencing partner abuse, what do you think might be the purpose of this behavior?

162 Virtual Clinical Excursions for Psychiatric Nursing

6. What is one of the most frightening realities that Dorothy Grant may face in leaving her husband?

7. Women in abusive relationships have characteristics in common. Knowing the characteristics that apply to Dorothy Grant will help the nurse in her assessment and interventions. Complete the table below by explaining how each of these general characteristics applies specifically to Dorothy Grant.

Common Characteristics of Women in Abusive Relationships	Dorothy Grant's Characteristics
Lack of relationships outside the home	
Inability to take action	
Internal feeling of emptiness	
Feeling of being disconnected	

8. Discharge planning is going to be crucial for Dorothy Grant. Which of the following activities will be necessary for a successful outcome? Select all that apply.

   _____ Creating a safety planning checklist

   _____ Providing access to other survivors of abuse and violence hotline phone numbers

   _____ Finding a supportive alternate living arrangement for her and her children

   _____ Referring her to legal assistance, financial aid, and job training and counseling

9. Do you believe that Dorothy Grant's current and past responses to the abuse are pathologic in nature, or do you think this is the typical way a person would react to physical and emotional trauma? Explain.

LESSON 14

The Adolescent Patient

Reading Assignment: Child and Adolescent Psychiatric Nursing (Chapter 40)

Patient: Tiffany Sheldon, Pediatrics Floor, Room 305

Goal: To provide psychiatric nursing care to an adolescent patient.

Objectives:

1. Understand factors involved in psychiatric disorders of adolescence.
2. Discuss the concept of resilience.
3. Identify key areas to include when assessing an adolescent patient.
4. Identify typical issues common in adolescence.
5. Explore unhealthy responses seen in adolescence.
6. Describe nursing interventions effective in working with adolescents.
7. Explore the nurse's own issues when working with adolescent patients.
8. Evaluate the nursing care for an adolescent patient.

Exercise 1

Writing Activity

15 minutes

1. Psychiatric disorders in adolescents are caused by an interaction of _____, _____, and _____ factors.

2. Discuss the concept of resilience and the role it plays in vulnerability to psychiatric disorders in adolescents.

3. Adolescents are concerned about many issues. What are some of the typical issues important to adolescents?

4. Body image, identity, and independence are three issues that can produce a variety of healthy and unhealthy responses as an adolescent attempts to cope with developmental tasks. Match each of these issues of adolescence with its corresponding characteristics.

Adolescent Issue

_____ Body image

_____ Identity

_____ Independence

Characteristics

a. Adolescents see themselves as being free of parental control. They often seek out adult situations and may become frightened and overwhelmed in the process.

b. Growth and development varies widely; growth is uneven and sudden; adolescents compare themselves with their peers.

c. Childhood dreams end. The adolescent often becomes negative and contrary; can feel isolated, lonely, and confused.

5. Unhealthy coping responses in adolescence include a variety of behaviors. Discuss the potentially unhealthy responses of adolescents to depression and body image distortion. (*Hint:* Feel free to draw from your own experiences.)

Exercise 2

 Virtual Hospital Activity

 45 minutes

- Sign in to work at Pacific View Regional Hospital on the Pediatrics Floor for Period of Care 3. (*Note:* If you are already in the virtual hospital from a previous exercise, click on **Leave the Floor** and then on **Restart the Program** to get to the sign-in window.)
- From the Patient List, select Tiffany Sheldon (Room 305).
- Click on **Go to Nurses' Station**.
- Click on **Chart** and then on **305**.
- Click on and review the **History and Physical**, **Nursing Admission**, and **Consultations** tabs.

1. In working with adolescents, the nurse must distinguish between age-expected behavior and unhealthy coping responses. For each adolescent age-expected behavior listed below, describe Tiffany Sheldon's corresponding unhealthy coping response.

Issue in Adolescence	Age-Expected Behavior	Tiffany Sheldon's Unhealthy Response
Body image	Focus is on weight, body image, and bodily sensation; compares self with others.	
Mood	Occasional and/or frequent sadness, worrying, moodiness, irritability.	
Activity	May vary between periods of sleep and high energy; may participate in school-related activities and sports; goal-directed activity can help with stress and excess energy.	

2. The specific problems of adolescence that make Tiffany Sheldon a high-risk adolescent are:
   a. substance use and truancy.
   b. severe eating disorder and depressed mood.
   c. suicidal and self-injurious behavior.
   d. problems with conduct and violence.
   e. anxiety and sexual promiscuity.

3. When working with adolescents, the nurse must understand a few basic principles. Which of the following statements best represent interventions the nurse can use when working with Tiffany Sheldon to demonstrate an understanding of these underlying principles? Select all that apply.

   _____ Use interventions that promote development of a trusting nurse-patient relationship.

   _____ Lecture Tiffany Sheldon on the importance of cooperating with the decisions her parents make.

   _____ Communicate empathy and understanding regarding the difficult developmental issues that Tiffany Sheldon is going through.

   _____ Role-model mature interpersonal relationships.

   _____ Only meet with Tiffany Sheldon together with her parents.

   _____ Maintain appropriate treatment boundaries.

   _____ Work to integrate the family's perspective with that of the adolescent.

4. Discuss the types of therapy suggested in the Psychiatric Consult to work with Tiffany Sheldon on the psychologic aspects of her unhealthy coping responses. Provide a possible rationale for each therapy. (*Hint:* Return to the Consultations in Tiffany Sheldon's chart if necessary.)

5. Discuss your own feelings about adolescence that might arise in working with a patient such as Tiffany Sheldon.

6. The nurse must objectively evaluate the nursing care that has been provided to Tiffany Sheldon and her family. Which of the following questions would be important to ask in determining whether Tiffany Sheldon and her family have met the treatment goals outlined in the treatment plan? Select all that apply.

   _____ Were Tiffany Sheldon's and her parents' concerns addressed?

   _____ Has Tiffany Sheldon's problematic behavior decreased and been replaced with more healthy coping responses?

   _____ Is Tiffany Sheldon at 100% of her normal body weight?

   _____ Have Tiffany Sheldon's activities of daily living become more reasonable in intensity?

   _____ Do Tiffany Sheldon and her family have a better understanding of her problems?

   _____ Are Tiffany Sheldon and her parents satisfied with the progress toward treatment goals?

   _____ Have Tiffany Sheldon's interpersonal relationships improved?

LESSON 15

Mental Disorders in Older Adults

Reading Assignment: Mental Disorders in Older Adults (Chapter 41)

Patient: Kathryn Doyle, Skilled Nursing Floor, Room 503

Goal: To understand, assess, and care for the older patient.

Objectives:

1. Identify factors in later life that contribute to good mental health.
2. Discuss ageism and how it impacts nursing care of the older patient.
3. Acknowledge personal biases in working with older adult patients.
4. Understand and use specialized knowledge and skills of the geropsychiatric nurse.
5. Identify components of a comprehensive assessment of an older patient.
6. Plan and coordinate the care for an older patient and her family.
7. Examine community aftercare support for the older adult patient and her family.

Exercise 1

Writing Activity

15 minutes

1. Mental health in later life depends on a number of factors. List several factors that can affect the mental health of the older adult.

2. Define *ageism* and discuss its implications for health care delivery. (*Hint:* Review ageist attitudes on page 469 of your textbook.)

3. Positive attitudes toward older adults and their care must be included in nursing education programs. Which of the following educational components should be included in a nursing education program? Select all that apply.

   _____ Information about the aging process

   _____ Discussion about nurses' attitudes toward working with older adults

   _____ Exploring the nurse-patient interactions with older adults

   _____ Teaching students how to develop sensitivity to the needs of older adults

4. In order to care effectively for older adult patients, the nurse needs to have specialized knowledge and skills. For each of the areas listed below, identify several skills the nurse must have in order to work with older patients.

Area	Specific Knowledge and Skills
Assessment	
Community resources	
Family and/or caregivers	
Medication	
Treatment modalities	
Advocacy	

5. Discuss possible biases you may have in working with older adults.

LESSON 15—MENTAL DISORDERS IN OLDER ADULTS   175

Exercise 2

 Virtual Hospital Activity

 45 minutes

- Sign in to work at Pacific View Regional Hospital on the Skilled Nursing Floor for Period of Care 2. (*Note:* If you are already in the virtual hospital from a previous exercise, click on **Leave the Floor** and then on **Restart the Program** to get to the sign-in window.)
- From the Patient List, select Kathryn Doyle (Room 503).
- Click on **Go to Nurses' Station**.
- Click on **Chart** and then on **503**.
- Click on and review the **Nursing Admission**, **History and Physical**, and **Consultations** tabs.

1. The four Ds of a comprehensive geriatric assessment are delirium, dementia, depression, and delusions. Depression is often confused with dementia and is not always recognized. Therefore the nurse needs to be familiar with the symptoms of later-life depression. According to the medical record, Kathryn Doyle has depression. What symptoms is Kathryn Doyle exhibiting that are consistent with later-life depression?

2. In addition to her depression, Kathryn Doyle also seems to be experiencing anxiety. Which of the following statements are true regarding anxiety in older adults? Select all that apply.

   _____ Comorbid anxiety and depression are common in older adults.

   _____ All types of anxiety combined are more prevalent than depression in older adults.

   _____ Untreated anxiety can contribute to sleep problems, cognitive impairments, and decreased quality of life.

   _____ Anxiety does not affect the family.

   _____ Antianxiety medications also decrease depression.

3. In addition to completing a mental status assessment, the nurse must include components specific to the nursing assessment of the older patient. Complete the table below to include information specific to Kathryn Doyle that corresponds with the key assessment elements identified.

Component	Key Assessment Elements	Corresponding Information from Kathryn Doyle's Assessment
Behavioral responses	Assess for problematic, disruptive, disturbing, or challenging behaviors occurring in the hospital, as well as those occurring where the patient lives; may be the first sign of many physical or mental health problems	
Functional abilities	Assessment of mobility and activities of daily living	
Physiologic responses	Assessment of physical health, nutrition, and medications, as well as substance abuse	
Social support	Assess support systems of the older patient because these are critical for maintaining a sense of well-being throughout life	

LESSON 15—MENTAL DISORDERS IN OLDER ADULTS   177

- Click on **Return to Nurses' Station**.
- Click on **MAR** and review Kathryn Doyle's medication list.

4. Does Kathryn Doyle have medication ordered to treat her depression? Discuss the role of medication to treat depression in the older adult.

5. Kathryn Doyle has many affective, somatic, stress, and behavioral issues common in older adults. For each issue listed below, briefly describe how the issue specifically affects Kathryn Doyle.

Issues Common in Older Adults	Kathryn Doyle's Situation
Situational low self-esteem	
Imbalanced nutrition	
Relocation stress syndrome	
Social isolation	

178 VIRTUAL CLINICAL EXCURSIONS FOR PSYCHIATRIC NURSING

- Click on **Return to Nurses' Station** and then on **503** at the bottom of the screen.
- Click on **Patient Care** and then on **Nurse-Client Interactions**.
- Select and view the video titled **1150: Depression—Cause, Treatment**. (*Note:* Check the virtual clock to see whether enough time has elapsed. You can use the fast-forward feature to advance the time by 2-minute intervals if the video is not yet available. Then click again on **Patient Care** and **Nurse-Client Interactions** to refresh the screen.)

6. Depression and sadness are sometimes viewed as a normal part of aging. Kathryn Doyle's responses to her life events of the past 9 months have resulted in a disturbance in her mood. List several events in Kathryn Doyle's recent history that have contributed to her depression.

- Click on **Leave the Floor** and then on **Restart the Program**.
- Sign in to work at Pacific View Regional Hospital on the Skilled Nursing Floor for Period of Care 3.
- From the Patient List, select Kathryn Doyle (Room 503).
- Click on **Go to Nurses' Station** and then on **503** at the bottom of the screen.
- Click on **Patient Care** and then on **Nurse-Client Interactions**.
- Select and view the video titled **1505: Assessment—Elder Abuse**. (*Note:* Check the virtual clock to see whether enough time has elapsed. You can use the fast-forward feature to advance the time by 2-minute intervals if the video is not yet available. Then click again on **Patient Care** and **Nurse-Client Interactions** to refresh the screen.)

7. Elder neglect and abuse has become more common in our society as older adults no longer have the status of respect they once had. Serving as Kathryn Doyle's advocate, the nurse must be alert for signs of elder neglect, abuse, or exploitation. What are the signs that Kathryn Doyle is being neglected, abused, or exploited?

8. In the family conference, the nurse will need to discuss whether or not Kathryn Doyle should continue to live in her son's home after she is discharged from the hospital. In order for the current living arrangement to work, the environment must include several basic characteristics appropriate for the older adult. Which of the following are critical elements you think should be included in Kathryn Doyle's home environment? Select all that apply.

   _____ Sense of calm and quiet

   _____ Structured routine, usual for her lifestyle

   _____ Consistent physical layout

   _____ Activities that produce cognitive stimulation

   _____ Safe environment

   _____ Personal items that provide familiarity and a sense of security

   _____ A focus on her strengths and abilities

9. About 80% of older adults are cared for in the home. What topics should the nurse include in family education and support sessions that would be critical to Kathryn Doyle's recovery and future?

10. Aftercare for older patients is often necessary for a successful treatment outcome. After discharge, what agency support do you think Kathryn Doyle's son will need in the care of his mother in the home?